THE POWER OF
GENUINELY CARING

DEDICATED TO MY READERS AROUND THE WORLD, MY HIGHER SELF, AND TO MY LOVING FRIENDS AND FAMILY

INTRODUCTION

Once upon a time in a small, tight-knit village nestled between rolling hills and lush forests, there lived a young woman named Elizabeth. Elizabeth was known for her warm heart and genuine care for everyone in her community. She always went out of her way to help others, whether it was tending to the sick, lending an ear to someone in distress, or simply sharing a smile and kind words.

One winter, the village was struck by a severe snowstorm. The roads were blocked, and supplies couldn't be delivered. The villagers were worried about running out of food and firewood, and many were trapped in their homes, struggling to stay warm.

Elizabeth, determined to help, rallied the villagers together. She organized a group of volunteers to check on every household, ensuring that everyone had enough provisions and warmth. Elizabeth herself visited the elderly and the sick, bringing them hot meals and firewood, and spending time with them to lift their spirits.

In one of her visits, she met an old man named Roderick. He lived alone and had always kept to himself, rarely interacting with others. Elizabeth discovered that Roderick had run out of firewood and was too weak to fetch more. She immediately brought him some from her own supply and stayed to prepare a meal for him. Over the next few days, Elizabeth visited Roderick regularly, learning about his life and sharing stories of the village.

Roderick, who had been lonely and withdrawn, slowly began to open up. He shared that he had once been a skilled carpenter but had stopped working after the death of his wife. Elizabeth encouraged him to reconnect with his passion, and with her support, Roderick decided to make small wooden toys for the village children.

As the storm subsided, the village came together to clear the roads and rebuild their lives. The children were delighted with Roderick's toys, and he found joy and purpose in his craft once more. The village, inspired by Elizabeth's selflessness, began to look out for one another more than ever before. They formed stronger bonds and created a supportive, caring community.

The rewards of Elizabeth's genuine care were manifold. The village thrived, not just in terms of material recovery but also in spirit and unity. Roderick, once isolated, became a beloved figure in the community, finding happiness and fulfillment in his work and relationships.

Elizabeth's story spread beyond the village, inspiring neighboring communities to foster kindness and support. She became a symbol of the power of genuine care, demonstrating that the rewards of caring for others extend far beyond immediate help—they create lasting bonds, bring joy and purpose, and build resilient, compassionate communities.

And so, the village continued to flourish, a testament to the profound impact that one person's genuine care can have on the lives of many. Elizabeth's legacy lived on, reminding everyone that the rewards of caring for others are not just in the act itself, but in the enduring connections and shared humanity it fosters.

CONTENTS

PART 1

UNDERSTANDING THE POWER

THE POWER

WHAT IS THIS POWER OF GENUINELY CARING FOR OTHERS ALL ABOUT?

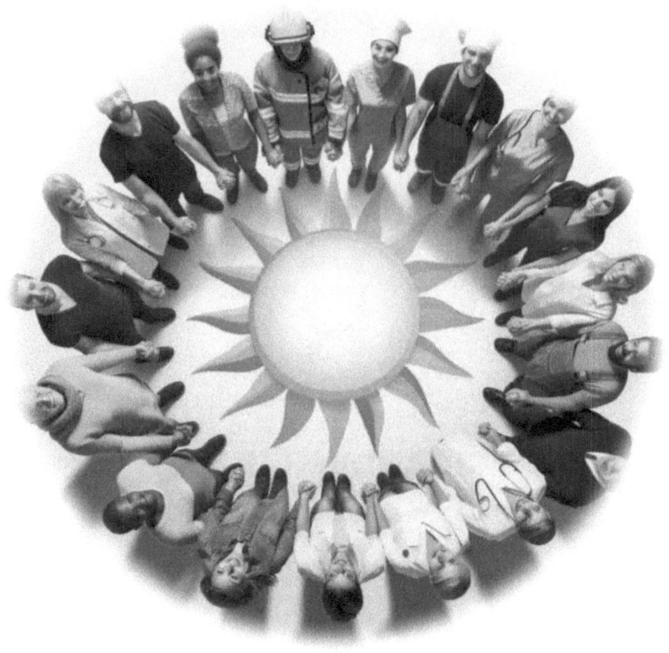

The power of genuinely caring for others lies in its ability to transform lives, foster strong and supportive communities, and drive positive social change. It enhances emotional and physical well-being, promotes social harmony, and inspires a culture of compassion. By embracing and practicing genuine care, we contribute to a more empathetic, just, and resilient world.

HOPE FOR THE WORLD

WHAT HOPE DOES THE WORLD HAVE FOR PEOPLE GENUINELY CARING ABOUT EACH OTHER?

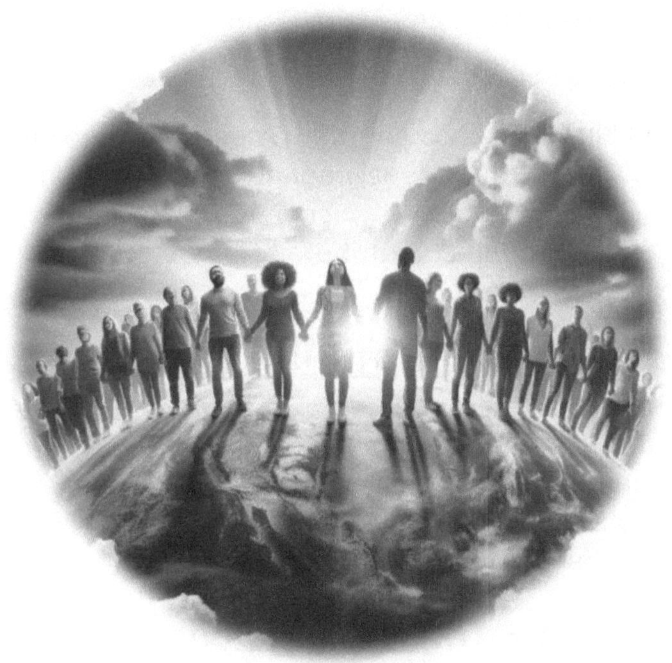

The world holds significant hope for people who genuinely care about each other, as these individuals and their actions contribute positively to various aspects of society and human well-being:

BUILDING STRONGER COMMUNITIES:

Genuine care fosters stronger social connections and community bonds. When people prioritize empathy and compassion, they create supportive environments where individuals feel valued and supported.

PROMOTING SOCIAL JUSTICE AND EQUALITY:

Caring about others often includes advocating for social justice, human rights, and equality. Individuals who genuinely care are more likely to take action against injustice and work towards creating a fairer and more inclusive society.

ENHANCING MENTAL AND EMOTIONAL WELL-BEING:

Acts of kindness and caring have been shown to improve mental health outcomes, reduce stress, and increase overall happiness. By supporting each other emotionally, people contribute to a healthier collective psyche.

FOSTERING GLOBAL COOPERATION:

Genuine care transcends cultural, ethnic, and national boundaries. It promotes understanding and collaboration across diverse communities, leading to greater global cooperation and harmony.

EMPOWERING INDIVIDUALS:

When individuals feel genuinely cared for, they are more likely to thrive and achieve their potential. Genuine care nurtures self-esteem, resilience, and a sense of belonging, empowering individuals to overcome challenges and pursue their goals.

CREATING LASTING IMPACT:

Small acts of kindness and caring can have ripple effects that create meaningful, long-lasting impact in communities and beyond. Whether through volunteering, mentoring, or advocacy, individuals who care genuinely contribute to positive change.

INSPIRING FUTURE GENERATIONS:

People who embody genuine care serve as role models for others, inspiring future generations to prioritize empathy, compassion, and social responsibility. This perpetuates a cycle of caring that strengthens communities over time.

RESPONDING TO GLOBAL CHALLENGES:

In times of crisis or uncertainty, genuine care becomes a vital resource for resilience and collective response. Whether facing natural disasters, health emergencies, or socioeconomic challenges, caring communities rally together to support those in need.

BUILDING TRUST AND RESILIENCE:

Trust is foundational to healthy relationships and societal cohesion. Genuine care builds trust among individuals and communities, fostering resilience in times of adversity and strengthening bonds during times of prosperity.

ENRICHING QUALITY OF LIFE:

Ultimately, genuine care enhances the overall quality of life for individuals and societies alike. It promotes a sense of purpose, fulfillment, and connection that transcends material wealth and status, contributing to a more meaningful existence for all.

In essence, the hope lies in the collective efforts of individuals who choose to prioritize empathy, kindness, and genuine care in their interactions and actions.

BEHAVIORS AND ATTITUDES

HOW DOES **NOT** GENUINELY CARING MANIFEST IN BEHAVIORS AND ATTITUDES?

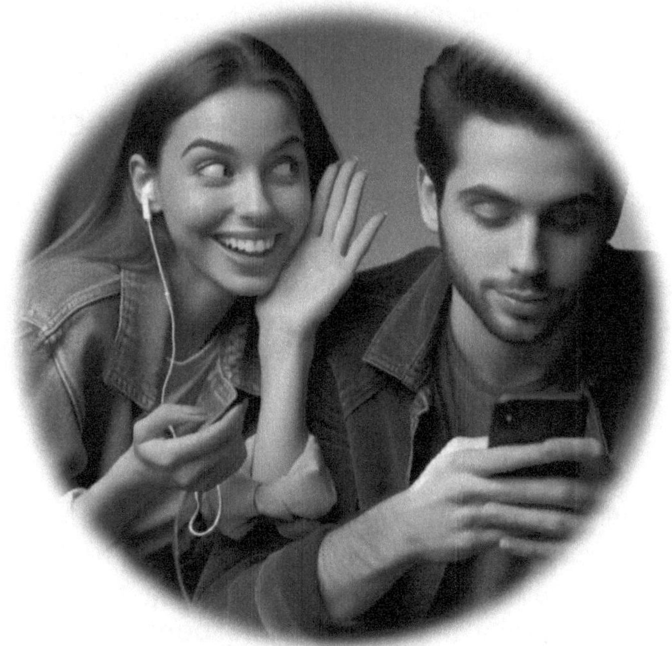

Not genuinely caring for others can manifest in various behaviors and attitudes. Here are some ways in which a lack of genuine care can be exhibited:

1. SUPERFICIAL CONCERN
2. MANIPULATIVE BEHAVIOR
3. SELF-CENTEREDNESS
4. INCONSISTENT AND UNRELIABLE BEHAVIOR
5. JUDGEMENTAL ATTITUDE
6. EXPOLITATIVE BEHAVIOR
7. EMOTIONAL DETACHMENT
8. PASSIVE-AGGRESSIVE BEHAVIOR
9. INAUTHENTIC BEHAVIOR
10. NEGLECTING SOCIAL RESPONSIBILITY

SUPERFICIAL CONCERN

- Fake Politeness: Displaying polite behavior without any real interest in the other person's well-being. This might involve saying things like "How are you?" without actually caring about the response.
- Pretending to Listen: Appearing to listen to someone while being distracted or disinterested. This can involve nodding or making generic responses without truly engaging in the conversation.

MANIPULATIVE BEHAVIOR

- Conditional Caring: Showing care and concern only when it benefits oneself, such as helping someone with the expectation of receiving something in return.
- Using Flattery: Giving insincere compliments or praise to manipulate others or gain favor, rather than out of genuine appreciation.

SELF-CENTEREDNESS

- Dominating Conversations: Focusing conversations on oneself and one's own experiences, showing little interest in hearing about others' lives or feelings.
- Ignoring Others' Needs: Failing to recognize or address the needs and feelings of others, prioritizing one's own desires and goals instead.

INCONSISTENT AND UNRELIABLE BEHAVIOR

- Breaking Promises: Frequently making promises or commitments and not following through, showing a lack of reliability and respect for others' trust.

- Being Unavailable: Regularly being emotionally or physically unavailable when others need support or assistance, indicating a lack of genuine care.

JUDGMENTAL ATTITUDE

- Criticizing Others: Being quick to judge or criticize others without offering constructive feedback or support, which can undermine trust and empathy.
- Showing Disdain or Condescension: Displaying a superior attitude or looking down on others, which can create emotional distance and hinder genuine caring.

EXPLOITATIVE BEHAVIOR

- Taking Advantage: Exploiting others for personal gain, whether emotionally, financially, or socially, without considering the impact on those being used.
- Lack of Reciprocity: Expecting others to be there for you while not being willing to reciprocate when they need support.

EMOTIONAL DETACHMENT

- Withholding Affection: Being emotionally distant or withholding affection and support, making others feel unimportant or unloved.
- Avoiding Emotional Intimacy: Avoiding deep and meaningful conversations or connections, keeping relationships at a superficial level.

PASSIVE-AGGRESSIVE BEHAVIOR

- Indirect Hostility: Expressing negative feelings indirectly through sarcasm, backhanded compliments, or other passive-aggressive behaviors rather than addressing issues openly and honestly.
- Sabotaging Efforts: Undermining others' efforts or achievements in subtle ways, indicating a lack of genuine support or care.

INAUTHENTIC BEHAVIOR

- Putting on a Facade: Acting in a way that is not true to oneself to manipulate others or create a false impression of caring.
- Insincere Apologies: Offering apologies that lack sincerity or are given only to avoid conflict rather than out of genuine remorse.

NEGLECTING SOCIAL RESPONSIBILITY

- Ignoring Social Cues: Failing to pick up on or respond to social cues that indicate someone needs support, showing a lack of social awareness and empathy.
- Failing to Act: Seeing someone in need and choosing not to help, whether out of indifference, laziness, or self-interest.

A lack of genuine care for others can manifest in superficial concern, manipulative behavior, self-centeredness, inconsistency, judgmental attitudes, exploitation, emotional detachment, passive-aggressiveness, inauthentic behavior, and neglecting social responsibility. These behaviors and attitudes undermine trust, empathy, and meaningful relationships, creating emotional distance and alienation.

BEHAVIORS AND ATTITUDES

WHAT ARE SOME OF THE MAIN BEHAVIORS AND ATTITUDES THAT REFLECT **GENUINELY CARING** ABOUT OTHERS?

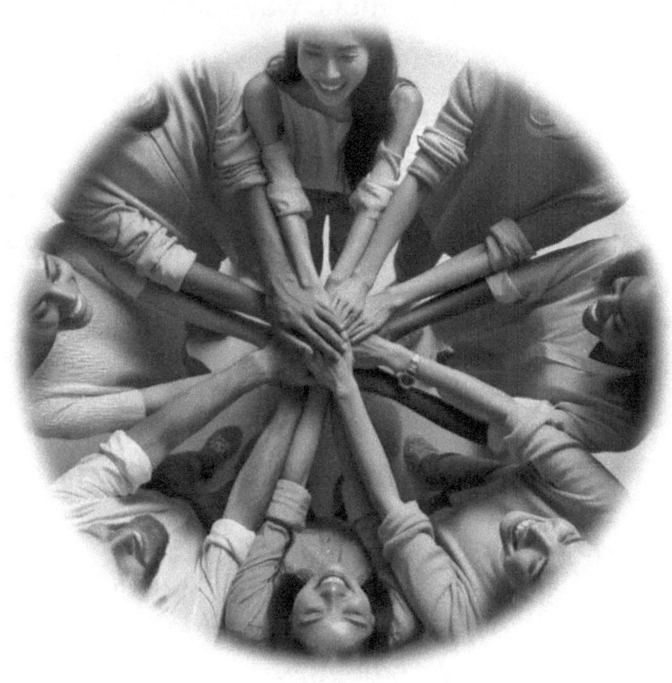

1. EMPATHY
2. RESPECT
3. AUTHENTICITY
4. ALTRUISM
5. RELIABILITY
6. SUPPORTIVENESS
7. HUMILITY
8. PATIENCE
9. COMPASSION
10. ENCOURAGEMENT

Genuinely caring about others involves specific behaviors and attitudes that reflect empathy, respect, and a sincere interest in their well-being. Here are the best behaviors and attitudes for demonstrating genuine care:

EMPATHY

- Active Listening: Give full attention when someone is speaking, show interest, and respond thoughtfully. Avoid interrupting and show understanding through nodding and verbal affirmations.
- Understanding Emotions: Try to understand and validate others' feelings and perspectives. Reflect back what you hear to ensure clarity and demonstrate empathy.

RESPECT

- Acknowledge Boundaries: Respect others' personal space, time, and boundaries. Avoid pushing people to share more than they are comfortable with.
- Show Appreciation: Regularly express gratitude and appreciation for others' efforts and presence. Acknowledge contributions and give credit where it is due.

AUTHENTICITY

- Be Genuine: Be sincere in your interactions and avoid putting on a facade. Share your true feelings and thoughts in a respectful manner.

- Honesty: Be truthful and transparent in your communication. Admit mistakes and apologize sincerely when necessary.

ALTRUISM

- Acts of Kindness: Perform selfless acts of kindness without expecting anything in return. Offer help and support whenever you see someone in need.
- Volunteering: Engage in community service or volunteer activities that help others. Dedicate time and effort to causes that benefit those in need.

RELIABILITY

- Keep Promises: Follow through on commitments and promises. Be dependable and consistent in your actions.
- Be Punctual: Respect others' time by being punctual and honoring appointments and deadlines.

SUPPORTIVENESS

- Offer Support: Provide emotional, practical, or financial support when someone is going through a tough time. Encourage and motivate others in their pursuits and challenges.
- Be Available: Make yourself available to listen and help when others reach out. Check in regularly with loved ones to show that you care.

HUMILITY

- Be Modest: Avoid bragging or seeking admiration. Acknowledge and appreciate the strengths and contributions of others.
- Admit Faults: Recognize and admit your mistakes. Learn from them and make efforts to improve.

PATIENCE

- Be Patient: Show patience when others are struggling or taking time to open up. Understand that everyone has their own pace and process.
- Avoid Judgment: Refrain from judging others harshly. Be open-minded and understanding of different perspectives and experiences.

COMPASSION

- Show Compassion: Express concern and empathy for others' suffering. Offer comfort and support to those in distress.
- Be Forgiving: Practice forgiveness and let go of grudges. Understand that everyone makes mistakes and deserves compassion.

ENCOURAGEMENT

- Positive Reinforcement: Encourage others with positive feedback and reinforcement. Celebrate their successes and milestones.
- Motivation: Help others find motivation and inspiration. Support their goals and aspirations with genuine enthusiasm.

The best behaviors and attitudes for genuinely caring about others include demonstrating empathy, respect, authenticity, altruism, reliability, supportiveness, humility, patience, compassion, and encouragement.

REFLECTION

WHAT ARE SOME OF OUR BEHAVIORS AND ATTITUDES IN GENUINELY CARING?

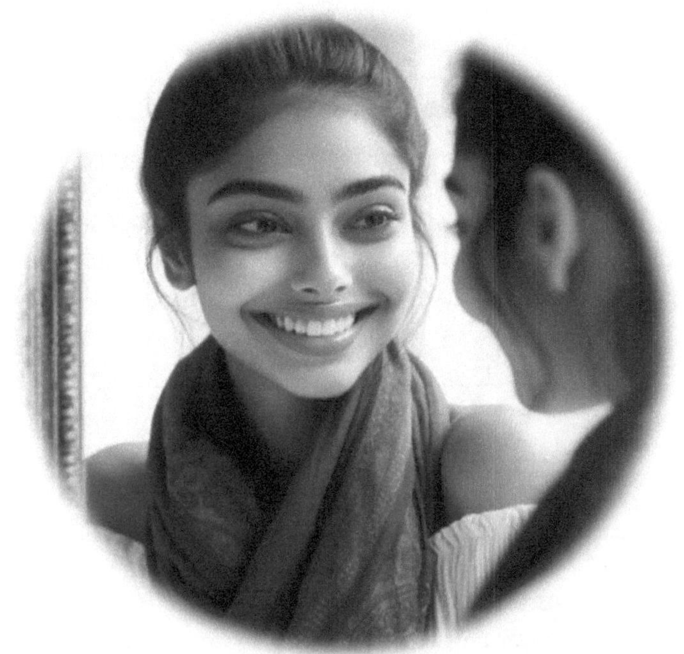

EXPLORING BEHAVIORS:

Reflect on a recent interaction where you felt disconnected or distant from someone. What were your behaviors in that situation?

____

____

____

Think about a time when you prioritized your own needs over someone else's. How did this affect your relationship with that person?

____

____

____

Describe a situation where you found it challenging to empathize with someone else's perspective or emotions. What barriers did you encounter?

____

____

____

Have you ever been accused of being manipulative or controlling in your interactions with others? Reflect on any instances and consider the impact on your relationships.

____

____

____

Think of a time when you were inconsistent or unreliable in your commitments to others. How did this affect trust and genuine care in those relationships?

____

____

____

EXAMINING ATTITUDES:

Consider your attitudes towards certain groups or individuals. Are there any prejudices or biases that influence how you interact with them?

____

____

____

Reflect on moments when you felt apathetic or indifferent towards someone's struggles or achievements. What underlying attitudes contributed to this response?

____

____

____

Have you ever engaged in relationships primarily for personal gain or utility? Reflect on how transactional attitudes may impact your ability to genuinely care for others.

____

____

____

Think about your typical response during conflicts or disagreements. Do you tend to respond with hostility, defensiveness, or avoidance? What beliefs or attitudes drive these responses?

____

____

____

Consider your level of empathy towards others. Reflect on any instances where you may have lacked empathy or struggled to understand someone's emotions. What attitudes or beliefs contributed to these challenges?

____

____

____

Reflect on situations where you've prioritized your own comfort or convenience over someone else's needs. How did this impact your relationship with that person?

____

____

____

Think about times when you've dismissed or minimized someone else's feelings or experiences. What motivated these responses?

____

____

____

Consider your willingness to offer emotional support to others. Reflect on any instances where you may have neglected to provide comfort or validation during challenging times.

____

____

____

GROWTH AND CHANGE:

What steps can you take to cultivate greater empathy and understanding towards others?

____

____

____

How can you become more aware of and address any biases or prejudices that may affect your interactions with others?

____

____

____

What strategies can you implement to build more trusting and supportive relationships based on genuine care and compassion?

____

____

____

Reflect on role models or individuals you admire for their ability to genuinely care for others. What qualities or behaviors can you emulate in your own life?

____

____

____

How can you practice more consistent and reliable behaviors in your relationships, ensuring that your actions align with your values of caring and empathy?

____

____

____

CHALLENGES

WHAT ARE <u>SOME OF THE CHALLENGES</u> WE FACE, WHEN WE START GENUINELY CARING?

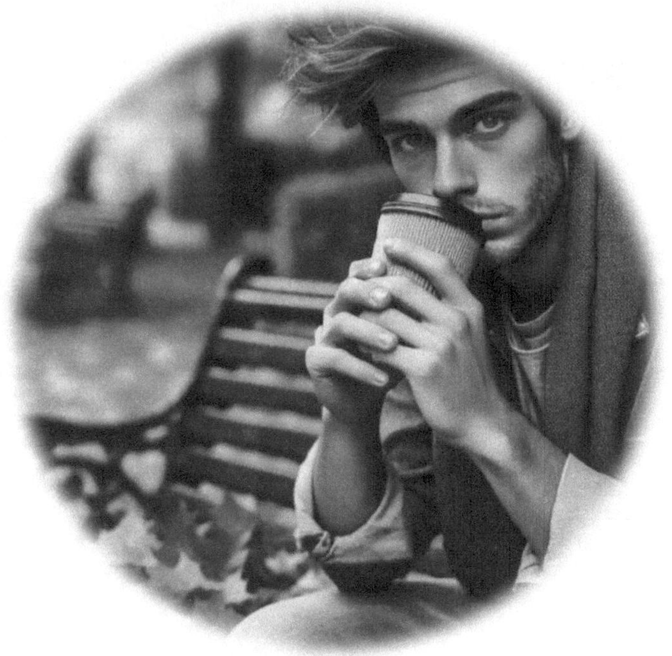

1. **EMOTIONAL DRAIN**
2. **BOUNDARIES**
3. **RECIPROCITY**
4. **VULNERABILITY**
5. **MISUNDERSTANDINGS**
6. **OVER-INVOLVEMENT**
7. **RESOURCE LIMITATION**
8. **EMOTIONAL BIAS**
9. **CONFLICTING NEEDS**
10. **PERSONAL GROWTH**

Genuinely caring about others can be deeply rewarding, but it also comes with several challenges:

EMOTIONAL DRAIN:

Consistently caring for others can be emotionally draining, especially if you're dealing with their problems and stresses regularly. This can lead to burnout and compassion fatigue.

BOUNDARIES:

Balancing care for others with personal boundaries can be difficult. Without clear boundaries, you might end up neglecting your own needs and well-being.

RECIPROCITY:

There is a risk that your care and kindness may not always be reciprocated, which can lead to feelings of frustration, resentment, or being taken for granted.

VULNERABILITY:

Genuinely caring about others often requires vulnerability. This can be challenging as it involves opening up and risking emotional hurt if the care is not returned or appreciated.

MISUNDERSTANDINGS:

Sometimes, genuine care can be misunderstood or misinterpreted. People might question your motives or think you have ulterior motives, which can strain relationships.

OVER-INVOLVEMENT:

There is a risk of becoming too involved in others' lives, which can lead to codependency or an inability to let them handle their own problems and growth.

RESOURCE LIMITATION:

Caring for others requires time, energy, and sometimes financial resources. Balancing these with your own responsibilities and resources can be challenging.

EMOTIONAL BIAS:

Genuine care can sometimes cloud judgment, making it difficult to remain objective or to make tough decisions that might be necessary.

CONFLICTING NEEDS:

Sometimes, genuinely caring for one person can put you in conflict with the needs or expectations of another, creating difficult choices and potential conflicts.

PERSONAL GROWTH:

Prioritizing others' needs might sometimes come at the expense of your own personal growth and development if not managed properly.

While these challenges are significant, they can be managed with self-awareness, effective boundary-setting, and self-care practices.

CHALLENGES

HOW DO WE <u>OVERCOME THE CHALLENGES</u> THAT DISCOURAGE US FROM GENUINELY CARING FOR OTHERS?

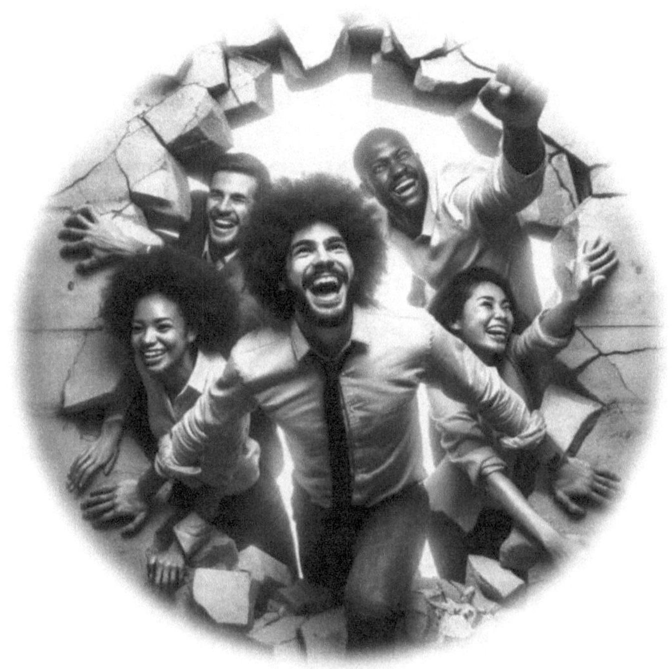

Overcoming the challenges of genuinely caring for others requires a combination of self-awareness, practical strategies, and support. Here are some effective ways to address these challenges:

TIME MANAGEMENT:

- Prioritize: Identify the most important tasks and focus on them.
- Schedule: Allocate specific times for caring activities to ensure they fit into your routine.
- Delegate: Share responsibilities with others when possible to balance your workload.

EMOTIONAL BURNOUT:

- Set Boundaries: Know your limits and communicate them clearly.
- Self-Care: Engage in activities that recharge you, such as exercise, hobbies, and relaxation techniques.
- Seek Support: Talk to friends, family, or a therapist about your feelings and challenges.

BALANCING PERSONAL NEEDS WITH CARING FOR OTHERS:

- Self-Reflection: Regularly assess your needs and ensure you are not neglecting them.
- Combine Activities: Find ways to integrate personal interests with caring activities (e.g., volunteering for causes you are passionate about).

FEELING OVERWHELMED:

- Break Tasks into Smaller Steps: Tackle one thing at a time to make the process more manageable.
- Set Realistic Goals: Understand that you cannot do everything and focus on achievable goals.
- Ask for Help: Don't hesitate to reach out to others for assistance.

DEALING WITH DIFFICULT SITUATIONS OR PEOPLE:

- Develop Empathy: Try to understand the other person's perspective and feelings.
- Stay Calm: Practice techniques to stay calm and composed during challenging interactions.
- Seek Mediation: In cases of conflict, consider involving a neutral third party to help mediate.

MAINTAINING GENUINE MOTIVATION:

- Remind Yourself of Your Purpose: Reflect on why you care for others and the positive impact it has.
- Celebrate Successes: Acknowledge and celebrate the positive outcomes of your efforts.
- Stay Connected: Surround yourself with like-minded individuals who share your values and goals.

LEARNING AND GROWING:

- Continual Learning: Engage in ongoing education about empathy, compassion, and effective caring strategies.
- Adaptability: Be open to changing your approach based on feedback and new insights.

RESOURCE LIMITATIONS:

- Use Available Resources Wisely: Make the most of what you have and seek out additional resources when needed.
- Collaborate: Work with others to pool resources and maximize impact.
- Advocate: Advocate for more resources and support within your community or organization.

By implementing these strategies, you can better manage the challenges associated with genuinely caring for others, ensuring that you remain effective, balanced, and fulfilled in your efforts.

WHAT DO WE NOW KNOW ABOUT OVERCOMING THE CHALLENGES OF GENUINELY CARING FOR OTHERS?

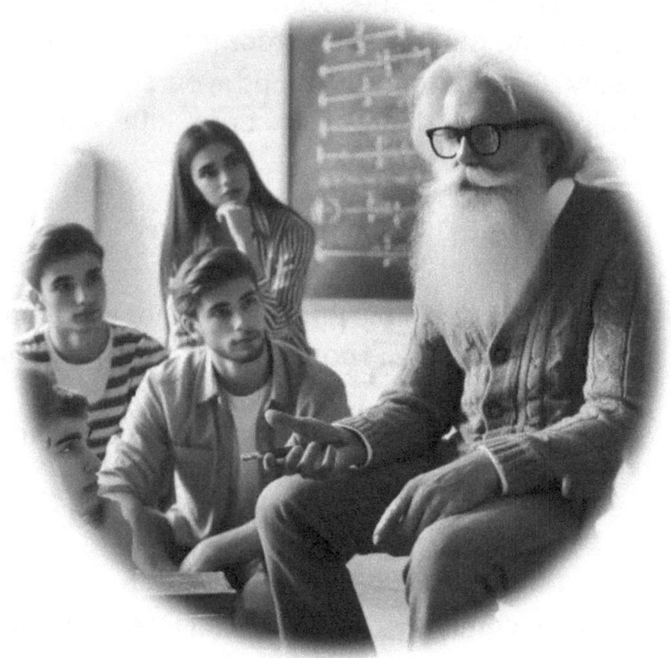

Quiz: Overcoming the Challenges of Genuinely Caring for Others

1. When someone shares a problem with you, your first instinct is to:

a) Offer immediate advice.

b) Listen carefully and empathize.

 c) Change the subject to something more positive.

d) Relate it to a similar problem you had.

2. How do you handle conflicts with others?

a) Avoid the person until things cool down.

b) Address the issue with empathy and understanding.

c) Defend your position strongly.

d) Try to find a quick compromise.

3. When you see someone in need of help, you:

a) Assume someone else will step in.

b) Offer assistance if you're not too busy.

c) Jump in to help immediately.

d) Wait to be asked before offering help.

4. How often do you practice active listening (listening without interrupting and with full attention)?

a) Rarely b) Sometimes c) Often d) Always

5. Reflecting on your own needs vs. others' needs, you typically:

a) Prioritize your needs first.

b) Balance your needs with others' needs.

c) Always put others' needs first.

d) Consider others' needs but often focus on your own.

6. How do you respond to others' emotions, especially when they are strong or negative?

a) I find it uncomfortable and try to change the subject.

b) I listen and try to understand their feelings.

c) I offer solutions to fix the problem.

d) I empathize but keep an emotional distance.

7. When a friend or family member is going through a tough time, you:

a) Send them a supportive message.

b) Spend time with them and offer your support.

c) Offer practical help (e.g., running errands, cooking).

d) Give them space to process on their own.

8. How do you react when someone disappoints you or makes a mistake?

a) I get frustrated and let them know.

b) I try to understand their perspective and forgive them.

c) I distance myself from them.

d) I quickly move on and don't dwell on it.

9. How comfortable are you with showing vulnerability to others?

a) Very uncomfortable

b) Somewhat uncomfortable

c) Comfortable

d) Very comfortable

10. How do you ensure you maintain your own well-being while caring for others?

a) I rarely think about my own well-being.

b) I balance my needs with others' needs.

c) I often neglect my own well-being.

d) I prioritize self-care to better support others.

Scoring:

- For each question, give yourself:
    - 1 point for each (a)
    - 2 points for each (b)
    - 3 points for each (c)
    - 4 points for each (d)

Results:

10-20 points: Growing Giver

You are beginning to navigate the challenges of caring for others but often find it difficult. Focus on listening and empathizing without immediately jumping to solutions. Practice small acts of kindness and consider others' perspectives.

21-30 points: Compassionate Companion

You show genuine care for others and balance your needs with theirs. Continue to practice active listening and empathy. Work on handling conflicts with understanding and maintaining your well-being.

31-40 points: Empathetic Ally

You are highly empathetic and often put others' needs first. Ensure you maintain your own well-being to avoid burnout. Encourage open communication and vulnerability in your relationships.

41-50 points: Caring Champion

You excel at genuinely caring for others and have mastered the balance between empathy and self-care. Continue to inspire others with your compassion and kindness and seek opportunities to mentor others in developing their caring abilities.

This quiz is designed to be both fun and insightful, helping you identify areas for growth and reinforcing the positive aspects of your caring nature.

CONSEQUENCES

WHAT ARE SOME OF THE <u>CONSEQUENCES</u> WE FACE WHEN WE STOP GENUINELY CARING?

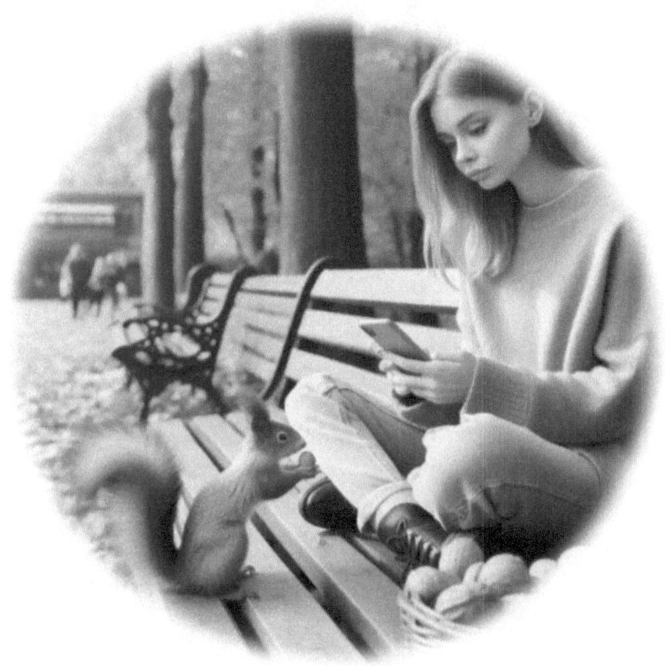

When people stop genuinely caring for others, several negative consequences can arise, impacting their personal well-being, relationships, and broader social dynamics. Here are some potential outcomes:

PERSONAL CONSEQUENCES:

- Emotional Isolation: Individuals may feel increasingly isolated and lonely as genuine connections with others diminish. Superficial relationships may lack the depth needed for emotional support and fulfillment.
- Increased Stress and Anxiety: Lack of meaningful interactions can lead to heightened stress and

anxiety. Caring for others often provides a sense of purpose and reduces stress; without it, individuals may feel more burdened by their own problems.

- Reduced Happiness and Life Satisfaction: Helping and caring for others often boosts happiness and life satisfaction. Without these positive interactions, individuals may experience a decline in overall happiness and fulfillment.
- Stagnation of Personal Growth: Genuine caring fosters empathy, compassion, and emotional intelligence. Without these experiences, personal growth and emotional development may stagnate.

RELATIONSHIP CONSEQUENCES:

- Weaker Relationships: Relationships may become strained or superficial without genuine care. Lack of empathy and support can lead to conflicts and misunderstandings.
- Loss of Trust: Trust is built through consistent, caring actions. Without genuine care, trust in personal and professional relationships may erode.
- Decreased Social Support: Individuals who do not care for others may find that others are less willing to support them in times of need. Reciprocity is a key aspect of social support networks.

SOCIAL CONSEQUENCES:

- Fragmented Communities: Communities rely on mutual support and cooperation to thrive. A lack of genuine care can lead to fragmented, less resilient communities.

- Increased Conflict and Tension: Empathy and understanding are crucial for resolving conflicts. Without genuine care, misunderstandings and conflicts may become more frequent and severe.
- Erosion of Social Cohesion: Social cohesion is strengthened by acts of care and kindness. Without these actions, societal bonds may weaken, leading to a more divided and less cooperative society.

BROADER IMPACTS:

- Decreased Overall Well-Being: Societal well-being is enhanced by a culture of caring and mutual support. A lack of genuine care can contribute to societal issues such as poor mental health, increased crime, and lower quality of life.
- Perpetuation of Social Inequality: Genuine care drives efforts to address social injustices and support marginalized individuals. Without it, social inequalities may persist or worsen, as fewer people advocate for change.
- Environmental Neglect: Genuine care often extends to the environment and other living beings. Without this care, environmental degradation and neglect of animal welfare are more likely.

PERSONAL AND PROFESSIONAL CONSEQUENCES:

- Professional Relationships: Lack of genuine care can impact professional relationships and workplace culture. Colleagues may be less likely to collaborate and support each other, affecting team dynamics and productivity.
- Career Impact: Caring behaviors can lead to networking opportunities and professional

growth. Without these behaviors, individuals may miss out on career advancements and opportunities.

In summary, when people stop genuinely caring for others, the negative impacts can be profound, affecting personal well-being, relationships, communities, and broader societal dynamics. Cultivating genuine care is essential for creating a supportive, thriving, and sustainable world.

REWARDS
WHAT ARE SOME OF THE REWARDS OF GENUINELY CARING ABOUT OTHERS?

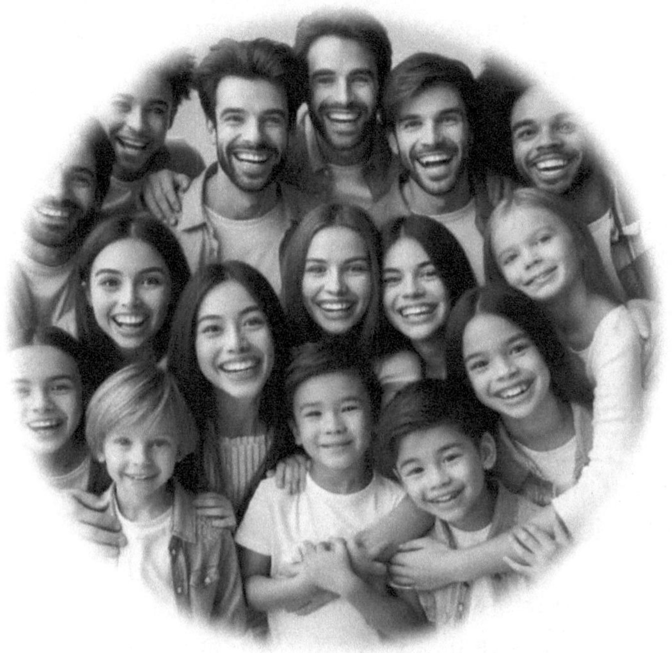

Genuinely caring about others can yield numerous rewards, both for the person showing care and for those on the receiving end. These rewards span emotional, social, physical, and psychological dimensions. Here are some of the key benefits:

EMOTIONAL REWARDS:

Increased Happiness: Engaging in acts of kindness and showing genuine care can boost your mood and overall sense of happiness. Positive interactions with others create feelings of joy and fulfillment.

Enhanced Empathy: By caring for others, you naturally become more attuned to their feelings and experiences, which can deepen your empathy and emotional intelligence.

Sense of Purpose: Caring for others provides a sense of meaning and purpose in life, as you contribute to the well-being and happiness of those around you.

Emotional Resilience: Building strong, supportive relationships through genuine care can enhance your emotional resilience, helping you cope with personal challenges and adversity.

SOCIAL REWARDS:

Strengthened Relationships: Genuine care fosters trust, mutual respect, and deeper connections in your relationships, leading to more meaningful and lasting bonds with others.

Social Support: By caring for others, you build a network of people who are likely to offer you support and care in return during times of need.

Positive Social Influence: Demonstrating genuine care can inspire others to act similarly, creating a ripple effect of kindness and compassion within your social circles and community.

Enhanced Reputation: Being known as a caring and compassionate person can positively impact your reputation, leading to greater respect and admiration from others.

PSYCHOLOGICAL REWARDS:

Improved Mental Health: Acts of kindness and showing care can reduce symptoms of depression, anxiety, and stress, contributing to overall mental well-being.

Increased Self-Esteem: Helping others and seeing the positive impact of your actions can boost your self-esteem and confidence.

Lower Stress Levels: Caring for others can lead to the release of stress-reducing hormones like oxytocin, promoting relaxation and well-being.

PHYSICAL REWARDS:

Better Physical Health: Studies have shown that people who engage in caring behaviors tend to have lower blood pressure, stronger immune systems, and reduced risk of chronic diseases.

Longevity: Engaging in positive social interactions and caring for others is associated with a longer lifespan, as social connections and altruism contribute to overall health and vitality.

SPIRITUAL AND ETHICAL REWARDS:

Spiritual Fulfillment: For many, caring for others aligns with their spiritual or religious beliefs, providing a sense of spiritual fulfillment and connection to a higher purpose.

Ethical Satisfaction: Acting with genuine care and compassion aligns with many ethical and moral frameworks, leading to a sense of integrity and ethical satisfaction.

PROFESSIONAL REWARDS:

Better Workplace Relationships: Demonstrating genuine care for colleagues can lead to a more positive and supportive work environment, enhancing teamwork and collaboration.

Leadership Opportunities: Leaders who show genuine care for their team members often inspire loyalty and higher performance, leading to greater professional success and leadership opportunities.

Career Satisfaction: Professionals in caregiving roles (e.g., healthcare, social work, education) often find deep satisfaction and fulfillment in their work through the genuine care they provide to others.

REFLECTIVE REWARDS:

Legacy Building: The care and compassion you show to others can create a lasting legacy, influencing how you are remembered and the positive impact you leave on the world.

Personal Growth: Engaging in genuine care encourages continuous personal growth, as you learn more about yourself and develop qualities like patience, understanding, and empathy.

The rewards of genuinely caring for others are profound and multifaceted, enriching your life and the lives of those around you. By fostering empathy, compassion, and genuine connections, you create a more positive and supportive environment, contributing to personal and collective well-being.

RESEARCH

WHAT **STUDIES** SHOW THE BENEFITS OF GENUINELY CARING ABOUT OTHERS?

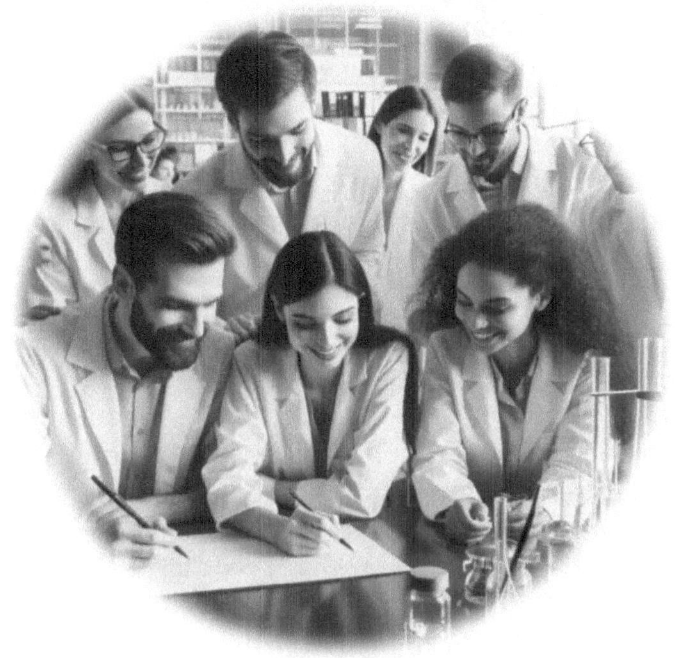

Several studies have examined the benefits of genuinely caring about others, demonstrating its positive impacts on various aspects of well-being and social dynamics. Here are some notable studies that highlight these benefits:

HEALTH BENEFITS:

Study: A meta-analysis by Post et al. (2019) reviewed multiple studies and found that engaging in prosocial behaviors, such as caring for others, is associated with reduced risk of mortality and improved physical health outcomes. These benefits were particularly pronounced in older adults.

MENTAL HEALTH AND HAPPINESS:

Study: Aknin et al. (2013) conducted research showing that spending money on others (prosocial spending) promotes happiness more than spending on oneself. This study demonstrated that acts of generosity and caring can enhance subjective well-being.

Study: Nelson et al. (2016) explored the psychological benefits of altruism and found that individuals who engage in regular acts of kindness report higher levels of life satisfaction and positive affect.

SOCIAL RELATIONSHIPS AND SUPPORT:

Study: Cacioppo & Patrick (2008) discussed the importance of social connections in promoting health and well-being. Genuine care and support from others contribute significantly to social capital and resilience in communities.

Study: Grant (2013) researched the impact of helping behaviors in workplace settings, finding that employees who engage in helping others experience greater job satisfaction and professional success due to improved relationships and collaboration.

LONGEVITY AND PHYSICAL HEALTH:

Study: Konrath et al. (2018) conducted longitudinal research showing that individuals who engage in regular volunteering and helping behaviors tend to live longer than those who do not. This study highlighted the protective effects of altruistic behaviors on physical health.

CHILDREN'S DEVELOPMENT:

Study: Eisenberg et al. (2015) explored the developmental benefits of empathy and caring behaviors in children. They found that children who are raised in nurturing environments with caregivers who model empathy are more likely to develop prosocial behaviors and emotional competence.

COMMUNITY AND SOCIETAL IMPACT:

Study: Putnam (2000) discussed the concept of social capital and its role in community well-being. Prosocial behaviors, including caring for others, contribute to the cohesion and resilience of communities, fostering a sense of collective responsibility and support.

These studies collectively illustrate that genuinely caring about others has profound positive effects on individual well-being, social relationships, community cohesion, and even physical health outcomes. They provide empirical evidence supporting the idea that altruistic behaviors not only benefit others but also enhance the giver's own happiness and overall quality of life.

<u>WHAT DO WE NOW KNOW</u> ABOUT THE REWARDS OF GENUINELY CARING?

QUIZ: DISCOVER THE REWARDS OF GENUINELY CARING FOR OTHERS

1. When you help someone in need, how does it make you feel?

a) Happy and fulfilled

b) Grateful and humbled

 c) Energized and motivated

d) Peaceful and content

2. What's the most noticeable change in your relationships when you show genuine care?

a) Deeper connections

b) Increased trust

c) Better communication

d) More mutual support

3. How has caring for others impacted your own mental health?

a) Reduced stress and anxiety

b) Increased happiness and joy

c) Enhanced sense of purpose

d) Greater emotional resilience

4. Which of these physical benefits have you experienced from caring for others?

a) Lower blood pressure

 b) Better overall health

c) Increased energy

d) Improved sleep

5. How does showing empathy and compassion affect your self-esteem?

a) Boosts my confidence

 b) Makes me feel valued

c) Encourages personal growth

d) Reinforces my sense of integrity

6. In what ways has your sense of community changed by genuinely caring for others?

a) Stronger social bonds

b) More collaborative efforts

c) Greater sense of belonging

d) Increased mutual respect

7. How do you feel after resolving a conflict with empathy and understanding?

a) Relieved and satisfied

b) Proud and accomplished

 c) Hopeful for the future

d) Closer to the other person

8. How does practicing genuine care influence your professional life?

a) Improved teamwork

b) Better leadership skills

c) Enhanced reputation

d) Greater job satisfaction

9. What spiritual or ethical rewards do you experience from caring for others?

a) Spiritual fulfillment

b) Ethical satisfaction

c) Sense of higher purpose

d) Alignment with personal values

10. How does showing care and compassion inspire those around you?

a) They become more empathetic

b) They engage in acts of kindness

c) They build stronger relationships

d) They create a supportive community

Scoring:

- For each question, give yourself:
    - 1 point for each (a)
    - 2 points for each (b)
    - 3 points for each (c)
    - 4 points for each (d)

Results:

10-20 points: Heartfelt Helper

You find joy and fulfillment in helping others, and it deeply impacts your emotional and physical well-being. Continue to nurture these feelings by engaging in acts of kindness and empathy.

21-30 points: Community Connector

Your genuine care strengthens your relationships and builds a sense of community. Embrace your role as a connector by fostering trust and collaboration among those around you.

31-40 points: Empathetic Influencer

You experience profound personal and professional growth through your caring nature. Leverage your empathy and leadership skills to inspire and support others in their journeys.

41-50 points: Compassionate Visionary

You embody the highest rewards of caring for others, including spiritual fulfillment and a strong sense of purpose. Use your compassionate vision to create positive change in your community and beyond.

PART 2

USING THE POWER ON PURPOSE

GENUINELY CARING

POWER #1 – **EMPATHY**

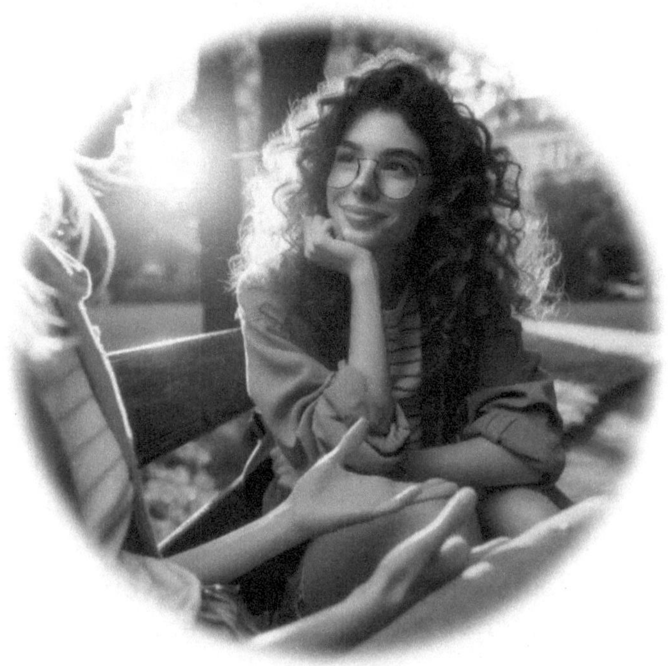

Developing empathy involves enhancing your ability to understand and share the feelings of others. Here are some effective ways to cultivate empathy:

ACTIVE LISTENING:

- Focus Fully: Pay close attention to what others are saying without interrupting.
- Reflect and Validate: Paraphrase what you've heard to show understanding and validate their feelings.

OBSERVE NONVERBAL CUES:

- Body Language: Notice gestures, facial expressions, and posture to understand unspoken emotions.
- Tone of Voice: Listen to the tone and pitch, which can convey feelings beyond words.

ENGAGE IN CONVERSATIONS:

- Ask Open-Ended Questions: Encourage others to share their thoughts and feelings more deeply.
- Show Genuine Curiosity: Be interested in their experiences and perspectives.

READ FICTION AND WATCH MOVIES:

- Diverse Stories: Engage with stories from different cultures and backgrounds to broaden your understanding of various perspectives.
- Character Analysis: Reflect on the emotions and motivations of characters to practice empathy.

PRACTICE MINDFULNESS:

- Stay Present: Focus on the present moment to better tune into others' feelings.
- Self-Awareness: Understand your own emotions and how they influence your reactions to others.

VOLUNTEER AND HELP OTHERS:

- Community Service: Engage in activities that involve helping people in different situations.
- Listen to Their Stories: Spend time understanding the challenges and experiences of those you help.

CULTIVATE CURIOSITY ABOUT OTHERS:

- Learn About Different Lifestyles: Take an interest in how others live, their traditions, and their values.
- Travel or Explore New Environments: Exposure to different cultures and communities can enhance empathy.

REFLECT ON PERSONAL EXPERIENCES:

- Recall Similar Situations: Think about times when you felt similar emotions to those being expressed by others.
- Journal Your Thoughts: Writing about your feelings and reactions can help you understand them better.

PRACTICE COMPASSIONATE RESPONSES:

- Acknowledge Emotions: Validate others' feelings even if you don't fully understand them.
- Offer Support: Show that you care through supportive words and actions.

LEARN FROM ROLE MODELS:

- Observe Empathetic People: Watch how empathetic individuals interact and respond to others.
- Seek Guidance: Ask for advice on developing empathy from those you admire.

TAKE PERSPECTIVE-TAKING EXERCISES:

- Put Yourself in Their Shoes: Imagine how you would feel in their situation.
- Role-Playing: Engage in exercises that require you to assume the perspective of others.

EDUCATE YOURSELF ON EMOTIONAL INTELLIGENCE:

- Read Books and Articles: Learn about empathy and emotional intelligence through various resources.
- Take Courses or Workshops: Participate in training that focuses on developing empathy and emotional skills.

Developing empathy is an ongoing process that involves continuous learning and practice. The more you practice these strategies, the better you will become at understanding and connecting with others on a deeper level.

WHAT EMPATHY STRATEGY OR STRATEGIES, SEEM MOST ATTRACTIVE TO **YOU** THAT WILL MAKE THE MOST IMPACT IN YOUR LIFE RIGHT NOW?

1.______________________________________

2.______________________________________

3.______________________________________

WHY WOULD THIS STRATEGY OR STRATEGIES MAKE THE MOST IMPACT IN YOUR LIFE RIGHT NOW?

1.______________________________________

____

WHAT **<u>STUDIES</u>** SHOW THE BENEFITS OF GENUINELY CARING FOR OTHERS USING EMPATHY?

Numerous studies highlight the benefits of genuinely caring for others through empathy, showing positive effects on mental health, relationship quality, and even physical health. Here are some key studies and findings:

EMPATHY AND MENTAL HEALTH:

A study published in the *Journal of Counseling Psychology* found that individuals who practice empathy experience lower levels of stress and anxiety. Empathy promotes emotional regulation and resilience, contributing to better mental health outcomes.

Another study in the *American Journal of Public Health* indicated that empathetic behavior can reduce symptoms of depression and improve overall life satisfaction. This study highlighted the role of social support and connectedness fostered by empathy.

EMPATHY AND RELATIONSHIP QUALITY:

Research published in the *Journal of Marriage and Family* showed that empathy is a critical factor in maintaining healthy romantic relationships. Partners who exhibit higher levels of empathy report greater relationship satisfaction, better communication, and increased emotional intimacy.

A study in *Child Development* found that empathetic parents have stronger bonds with their children. Children of empathetic parents demonstrate higher emotional intelligence, better social skills, and lower instances of behavioral problems.

EMPATHY AND PHYSICAL HEALTH:

The *American Journal of Medicine* published a study linking empathy in healthcare providers to improved patient outcomes. Patients with empathetic doctors report higher satisfaction levels, better adherence to treatment plans, and faster recovery times.

Another study in *Health Psychology* found that practicing empathy can boost immune function and reduce inflammation, suggesting a direct connection between emotional well-being and physical health.

EMPATHY AND WORKPLACE ENVIRONMENT:

Research in the *Journal of Applied Psychology* demonstrated that empathetic leaders create more positive work environments. Employees with empathetic managers experience lower levels of burnout, higher job satisfaction, and greater productivity.

A study in the *Harvard Business Review* reported that empathy in the workplace leads to better teamwork and collaboration. Organizations that prioritize empathy see increased innovation and improved employee morale.

EMPATHY AND PROSOCIAL BEHAVIOR:

A study published in *Personality and Social Psychology Bulletin* showed that empathy encourages prosocial behavior, such as helping, sharing, and volunteering. Individuals who exhibit empathy are more likely to engage in acts of kindness and contribute to the well-being of others.

Another study in *Social Cognitive and Affective Neuroscience* found that empathy activates brain regions associated with reward and pleasure, suggesting that caring for others can be intrinsically rewarding and fulfilling.

These studies collectively highlight the profound benefits of empathy, demonstrating its importance in fostering mental and physical health, enhancing relationships, and creating supportive communities and workplaces.

<u>WHAT DO WE NOW KNOW</u> ABOUT GENUINELY CARING USING EMPATHY?

EMPATHY AND CARING QUIZ

Instructions: For each question, choose the option that best describes your typical behavior. At the end, tally your points to see how empathetic and caring you are!

1. **When a friend shares a problem with you, you:**
   - A. Immediately give advice. (1 point)
   - B. Listen carefully and then offer support. (3 points)
   - C. Change the topic to lighten the mood. (0 points)
2. **If you see a stranger struggling to carry heavy bags, you:**
   - A. Offer to help them carry the bags. (3 points)
   - B. Ignore them and continue with your day. (0 points)
   - C. Feel bad for them but don't take any action. (1 point)
3. **When someone tells you about their achievement, you:**
   - A. Congratulate them and ask more about it. (3 points)
   - B. Mention a similar achievement of your own. (1 point)
   - C. Nod and quickly change the subject. (0 points)
4. **In a group conversation, you:**
   - A. Make sure everyone has a chance to speak. (3 points)
   - B. Talk the most and dominate the conversation. (0 points)

- o C. Listen but don't actively engage others. (1 point)

5. **When you notice a colleague is unusually quiet, you:**
   - o A. Ask them if everything is okay. (3 points)
   - o B. Assume they just want to be left alone. (1 point)
   - o C. Don't pay much attention to it. (0 points)

6. **How often do you engage in volunteer work or community service?**
   - o A. Regularly. (3 points)
   - o B. Occasionally. (1 point)
   - o C. Never. (0 points)

7. **If you overhear someone being teased or bullied, you:**
   - o A. Step in and defend them. (3 points)
   - o B. Feel bad but don't intervene. (1 point)
   - o C. Ignore it and walk away. (0 points)

8. **When a friend is upset, you:**
   - o A. Offer a listening ear and comfort them. (3 points)
   - o B. Give them space and avoid the situation. (0 points)
   - o C. Tell them to cheer up and move on. (1 point)

9. **When you hear about a disaster affecting people in another country, you:**
   - o A. Donate to relief efforts or raise awareness. (3 points)
   - o B. Feel sad but don't take any action. (1 point)
   - o C. Think it's not your problem. (0 points)

10. **How do you react when you see someone crying in public?**

- o A. Approach them and ask if they need help. (3 points)
- o B. Feel awkward and avoid them. (0 points)
- o C. Watch from a distance but don't engage. (1 point)

Scoring:

- **24-30 points**: You are highly empathetic and genuinely care for others. Keep up the great work!
- **16-23 points**: You show a good level of empathy but there's room for improvement. Try to be more proactive in showing care.
- **8-15 points**: You have some empathy but often miss opportunities to show it. Focus on listening and supporting others more.
- **0-7 points**: Empathy is not your strong suit. Consider working on understanding and connecting with others more deeply.

Reflection: Based on your score, think about areas where you can improve your empathy and caring behaviors. Consider practicing active listening, engaging more in community service, or simply being more present for those around you.

GENUINELY CARING

POWER #2 – **RESPECT**

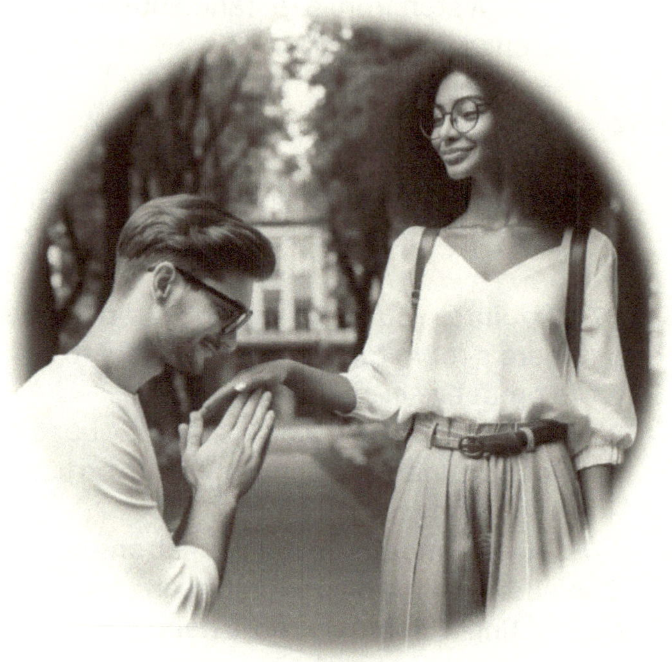

Developing respect involves cultivating attitudes and behaviors that recognize the value and dignity of others. Here are some effective ways to develop and demonstrate respect:

PRACTICE ACTIVE LISTENING:

- Give Full Attention: Focus on the speaker without interrupting or planning your response while they're talking.
- Show Interest: Use non-verbal cues like nodding and maintaining eye contact to show that you're engaged.

ACKNOWLEDGE DIFFERENCES:

- Embrace Diversity: Recognize and appreciate the differences in backgrounds, cultures, and perspectives.
- Avoid Stereotyping: Treat each person as an individual rather than making assumptions based on group characteristics.

SHOW COURTESY AND POLITENESS:

- Use Manners: Simple gestures like saying "please," "thank you," and "excuse me" go a long way.
- Be Punctual: Respect others' time by being on time for appointments and meetings.

VALUE OTHERS' OPINIONS:

- Be Open-Minded: Listen to and consider others' viewpoints, even if they differ from your own.
- Engage in Constructive Dialogue: Discuss differing opinions respectfully without dismissing or belittling them.

OFFER HELP AND SUPPORT:

- Be Considerate: Offer assistance when you see someone in need or struggling.
- Be Willing to Share: Share your knowledge, resources, and time generously.

RESPECT BOUNDARIES:

- Understand Limits: Be aware of personal and professional boundaries and respect them.
- Seek Consent: Always ask for permission before using someone's belongings or personal space.

ACKNOWLEDGE AND APOLOGIZE FOR MISTAKES:

- Own Your Actions: Take responsibility when you make a mistake and apologize sincerely.
- Learn and Improve: Use feedback and mistakes as opportunities to grow and improve your behavior.

SHOW APPRECIATION:

- Express Gratitude: Regularly thank people for their help and contributions.
- Recognize Efforts: Acknowledge and appreciate the efforts and achievements of others.

BE HONEST AND TRANSPARENT:

- Communicate Openly: Be honest in your interactions and avoid deceit.
- Build Trust: Consistently demonstrate reliability and integrity.

AVOID JUDGMENT AND CRITICISM:

- Be Understanding: Approach others with empathy and try to understand their situations and choices.
- Provide Constructive Feedback: Offer feedback that is helpful and encouraging rather than harsh or critical.

MAINTAIN HUMILITY:

- Recognize Your Limits: Acknowledge that you don't know everything and can learn from others.
- Value Others' Contributions: Appreciate and credit others' contributions and successes.

- Involve Everyone: Ensure that all voices are heard and valued in group settings.
- Create a Welcoming Environment: Foster a sense of belonging and acceptance for everyone.

Respect is built through consistent actions and attitudes that honor the value and dignity of others. By practicing these behaviors, you can develop deeper, more meaningful relationships and contribute positively to your community and environment.

WHAT RESPECT STRATEGY OR STRATEGIES, SEEM MOST ATTRACTIVE TO **YOU** THAT WILL MAKE THE MOST IMPACT IN YOUR LIFE RIGHT NOW?

1.______________________________________

2.______________________________________

3.______________________________________

WHY WOULD THIS STRATEGY OR STRATEGIES MAKE THE MOST IMPACT IN YOUR LIFE RIGHT NOW?

1.______________________________________

____

WHAT **STUDIES** SHOW THE BENEFITS OF GENUINELY CARING FOR OTHERS USING RESPECT?

Numerous studies highlight the benefits of genuinely caring for others using respect, demonstrating positive impacts on mental health, relationship quality, organizational performance, and societal well-being. Here are some key studies and findings:

RESPECT AND MENTAL HEALTH:

A study published in the *Journal of Counseling Psychology* found that individuals who feel respected by others experience lower levels of stress and anxiety. Respectful interactions promote a sense of security and self-worth, which contributes to better mental health outcomes.

Research in the *Journal of Applied Social Psychology* demonstrated that giving and receiving respect in relationships is linked to higher self-esteem and overall life satisfaction. Respectful behavior fosters positive self-regard and emotional well-being.

RESPECT AND RELATIONSHIP QUALITY:

A study in the *Journal of Marriage and Family* showed that mutual respect is a crucial factor in maintaining healthy and satisfying romantic relationships. Couples who practice respect experience better communication, trust, and emotional intimacy.

Research published in *Child Development* found that respect between parents and children leads to stronger family bonds and better developmental outcomes for children. Respectful parenting practices are associated with higher emotional intelligence and social competence in children.

RESPECT IN THE WORKPLACE:

A study in the *Harvard Business Review* reported that respect in the workplace leads to higher job satisfaction, increased engagement, and lower turnover rates. Employees who feel respected by their managers and colleagues are more motivated and committed to their work.

Research published in the *Journal of Organizational Behavior* found that respectful treatment in the workplace enhances teamwork, collaboration, and overall organizational performance. Respectful interactions create a positive work environment and foster a culture of mutual support and cooperation.

RESPECT AND SOCIAL BEHAVIOR:

A study in the *Journal of Social Psychology* demonstrated that respect fosters prosocial behavior, such as helping, sharing, and volunteering. Individuals who practice and receive respect are more likely to engage in actions that benefit others and their communities.

Research in *Social Psychological and Personality Science* found that respect promotes social cohesion and reduces instances of conflict and aggression. Societies that emphasize respect experience greater harmony and cooperation among their members.

RESPECT AND PHYSICAL HEALTH:

A study published in *Health Psychology* showed that respectful relationships contribute to better physical health outcomes. Individuals in respectful relationships have lower levels of stress-related health problems and better overall health.

Research in the *Journal of Behavioral Medicine* found that respect and positive social interactions boost immune function and reduce inflammation, highlighting the connection between respectful relationships and physical well-being.

These studies collectively highlight the significant benefits of genuinely caring for others using respect, demonstrating its importance in fostering mental and physical health, enhancing relationship quality, improving workplace dynamics, and promoting social harmony. By practicing respect in various aspects of life, individuals and communities can experience profound positive outcomes.

<u>WHAT DO WE NOW KNOW</u> ABOUT GENUINELY CARING USING RESPECT?

RESPECT AND CARING QUIZ

Instructions: For each question, choose the option that best describes your typical behavior. At the end, tally your points to see how respectful and caring you are!

1. **When someone shares their opinion, especially if it differs from yours, you:**
   - A. Listen attentively and consider their viewpoint. (3 points)
   - B. Interrupt to share your own opinion. (1 point)
   - C. Dismiss their opinion as wrong. (0 points)
2. **If you accidentally bump into someone, you:**
   - A. Apologize sincerely and check if they're okay. (3 points)
   - B. Say a quick "sorry" and move on. (1 point)
   - C. Ignore it and keep walking. (0 points)
3. **When you notice a new colleague at work, you:**
   - A. Introduce yourself and offer help if they need anything. (3 points)
   - B. Wait for them to approach you first. (1 point)
   - C. Ignore them and stick to your usual group. (0 points)
4. **During a group project, you:**
   - A. Ensure everyone has a chance to contribute and speak. (3 points)
   - B. Focus mainly on your own part and let others handle their own. (1 point)

- o   C. Take control and make all the decisions. (0 points)
5. **If a friend confides in you about a personal issue, you:**
    - o   A. Listen without judgment and offer support. (3 points)
    - o   B. Offer advice based on your own experiences. (1 point)
    - o   C. Change the subject to something lighter. (0 points)
6. **When you see someone being treated unfairly, you:**
    - o   A. Stand up for them and speak out against the unfair treatment. (3 points)
    - o   B. Feel bad but don't get involved. (1 point)
    - o   C. Stay out of it; it's not your problem. (0 points)
7. **How do you handle conflicts with others?**
    - o   A. Address the issue respectfully and seek a solution together. (3 points)
    - o   B. Avoid the person until things calm down. (1 point)
    - o   C. Get defensive and argue your point. (0 points)
8. **When someone asks for feedback on something they've done, you:**
    - o   A. Provide honest and constructive feedback. (3 points)
    - o   B. Give general feedback to avoid any conflict. (1 point)
    - o   C. Criticize them bluntly. (0 points)
9. **If a family member has different beliefs than you, you:**
    - o   A. Respect their beliefs and try to understand their perspective. (3 points)

- ○ B. Avoid discussing those topics with them. (1 point)
  - ○ C. Argue with them to change their mind. (0 points)
10. **When you make a mistake, you:**
  - ○ A. Admit it, apologize, and try to make amends. (3 points)
  - ○ B. Downplay it and move on quickly. (1 point)
  - ○ C. Deny it or blame someone else. (0 points)

Scoring:

- **24-30 points**: You are highly respectful and genuinely care for others. Keep up the great work!
- **16-23 points**: You show a good level of respect but there's room for improvement. Focus on being more considerate in challenging situations.
- **8-15 points**: You have some respect for others but often miss opportunities to show it. Try to be more mindful of your actions and their impact on others.
- **0-7 points**: Respect is not your strong suit. Consider working on understanding and valuing others more deeply.

Reflection: Based on your score, think about areas where you can improve your respect and caring behaviors. Consider practicing active listening, being more inclusive, and addressing conflicts with understanding and empathy. Respect is foundational to healthy relationships and communities, so cultivating it benefits everyone.

GENUINELY CARING

POWER #3 – **AUTHENTICITY**

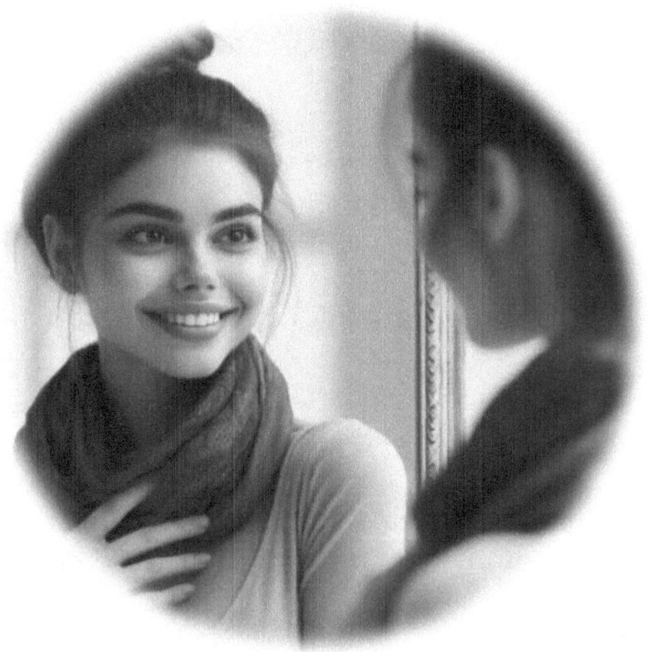

Developing authenticity involves being true to yourself, aligning your actions with your values, and being genuine in your interactions. Here are some effective ways to cultivate authenticity:

SELF-REFLECTION:

- Identify Your Values: Spend time understanding what truly matters to you and what you stand for.
- Reflect on Your Actions: Regularly assess if your behaviors and decisions align with your core values and beliefs.

EMBRACE VULNERABILITY:

- Be Open: Share your true thoughts and feelings with others, even if it feels uncomfortable.
- Accept Imperfections: Recognize that everyone has flaws and that it's okay to show them.

SET BOUNDARIES:

- Know Your Limits: Understand what you are comfortable with and what you are not.
- Communicate Clearly: Express your boundaries to others in a respectful and assertive manner.

PRACTICE SELF-COMPASSION:

- Be Kind to Yourself: Treat yourself with the same kindness and understanding that you would offer a friend.
- Forgive Yourself: Acknowledge your mistakes and learn from them without harsh self-criticism.

BE HONEST:

- Speak the Truth: Communicate honestly and transparently in your interactions.
- Avoid Pretense: Resist the urge to put on a façade to impress others or fit in.

FOLLOW YOUR PASSIONS:

- Pursue What You Love: Engage in activities and hobbies that genuinely interest you and bring you joy.
- Stay True to Your Interests: Don't let societal pressures or others' expectations deter you from your passions.

SURROUND YOURSELF WITH SUPPORTIVE PEOPLE:

- Choose Positive Relationships: Build relationships with people who accept and encourage your true self.
- Avoid Toxic Influences: Distance yourself from those who undermine your authenticity or pressure you to conform.

LISTEN TO YOUR INNER VOICE:

- Trust Your Intuition: Pay attention to your gut feelings and inner guidance.
- Make Decisions Based on Your Own Beliefs: Avoid making choices solely to please others or to gain approval.

BE CONSISTENT:

- Align Actions with Words: Ensure that your actions consistently reflect your spoken values and beliefs.
- Stay True in Different Situations: Maintain your authenticity regardless of the social context or pressures.

ACCEPT AND CELEBRATE YOUR UNIQUE IDENTITY:

- Embrace Your Uniqueness: Recognize and appreciate what makes you different from others.
- Share Your True Self: Don't be afraid to let others see your authentic personality and quirks.

DEVELOP EMOTIONAL AWARENESS:

- Understand Your Emotions: Regularly check in with your feelings and understand what they're telling you.
- Express Emotions Honestly: Share your true emotions with others, rather than hiding them.

PRACTICE MINDFULNESS:

- Stay Present: Focus on the present moment and be aware of your true self.
- Avoid Overthinking: Let go of excessive worries about others' perceptions or future outcomes.

Authenticity is about being genuine and true to yourself. By practicing these strategies, you can develop a deeper understanding of yourself and create more meaningful, authentic connections with others.

WHAT AUTHENTICITY STRATEGY OR STRATEGIES SEEM MOST ATTRACTIVE TO **YOU** THAT WILL MAKE THE MOST IMPACT IN YOUR LIFE RIGHT NOW?

1.____

2.____

3.____

WHY WOULD THIS STRATEGY OR STRATEGIES MAKE THE MOST IMPACT IN YOUR LIFE RIGHT NOW?

1.____

____

WHAT **STUDIES** SHOW THE BENEFITS OF GENUINELY CARING FOR OTHERS USING AUTHENTICITY?

Numerous studies highlight the benefits of genuinely caring for others using authenticity, demonstrating positive impacts on mental health, relationship quality, workplace dynamics, and overall well-being. Here are some key studies and findings:

AUTHENTICITY AND MENTAL HEALTH:

A study published in the *Journal of Counseling Psychology* found that authenticity is positively correlated with psychological well-being. Individuals who act in ways that are true to themselves experience lower levels of anxiety and depression and higher levels of life satisfaction.

Research in the *Journal of Personality and Social Psychology* showed that people who are authentic tend to have higher self-esteem and a greater sense of purpose in life. Being true to oneself reduces internal conflict and enhances overall mental health.

AUTHENTICITY AND RELATIONSHIP QUALITY:

A study in the *Journal of Social and Personal Relationships* indicated that authenticity in romantic relationships leads to greater relationship satisfaction and emotional intimacy. Partners who are genuine with each other experience more trust and a deeper connection.

Research published in *Personal Relationships* found that authentic self-disclosure is crucial for developing close and supportive friendships. Friends who share their true thoughts and feelings build stronger and more meaningful bonds.

AUTHENTICITY IN THE WORKPLACE:

A study in the *Journal of Applied Psychology* reported that authentic leadership leads to higher employee satisfaction and engagement. Leaders who are genuine and transparent inspire trust and loyalty among their team members.

Research in the *Journal of Business Ethics* found that employees who feel they can be authentic at work experience less burnout and higher job satisfaction. Authentic workplaces foster a positive organizational culture and enhance employee well-being.

AUTHENTICITY AND SOCIAL BEHAVIOR:

A study published in *Social Psychological and Personality Science* showed that authenticity promotes prosocial behavior. Individuals who are true to themselves are more likely to engage in helping behaviors and show compassion towards others.

Research in *Personality and Individual Differences* found that authenticity is associated with greater empathy and altruism. Being authentic helps individuals connect with others on a deeper level and understand their emotions and needs.

AUTHENTICITY AND PHYSICAL HEALTH:

A study in the *Journal of Health Psychology* demonstrated that authenticity is linked to better physical health outcomes. Individuals who live authentically report fewer stress-related health problems and better overall health.

Research in *Psychosomatic Medicine* found that authenticity can boost immune function and reduce the risk of chronic illnesses. Living in alignment with one's true self promotes physical well-being and resilience.

AUTHENTICITY AND OVERALL WELL-BEING:

A study in the *Journal of Positive Psychology* showed that authenticity contributes to greater overall well-being and happiness. People who are authentic experience more positive emotions and a greater sense of fulfillment in life.

Research published in *Self and Identity* found that authenticity enhances resilience and the ability to cope with life's challenges. Being true to oneself provides a stable foundation for navigating stress and adversity.

These studies collectively highlight the significant benefits of genuinely caring for others using authenticity, demonstrating its importance in fostering mental and physical health, enhancing relationship quality, improving workplace dynamics, and promoting overall well-being. By practicing authenticity in various aspects of life, individuals can experience profound positive outcomes and create more meaningful connections with others.

<u>WHAT DO WE NOW KNOW</u> ABOUT GENUINELY CARING USING AUTHENTICITY?

AUTHENTICITY AND CARING QUIZ

Instructions: For each question, choose the option that best describes your typical behavior. At the end, tally your points to see how authentic and caring you are!

1. **When a friend asks for your opinion, you:**
   - A. Share your honest thoughts, even if they differ from theirs. (3 points)
   - B. Sugarcoat your opinion to avoid hurting their feelings. (1 point)
   - C. Say what you think they want to hear. (0 points)

2. **In a group conversation, you:**
   - A. Express your true thoughts and feelings, even if they're different. (3 points)
   - B. Stay quiet and go along with the majority. (1 point)
   - C. Agree with everything to avoid conflict. (0 points)

3. **If you make a mistake at work, you:**
   - A. Admit it, apologize, and work to fix it. (3 points)
   - B. Try to downplay it and hope no one notices. (1 point)
   - C. Blame someone else to avoid repercussions. (0 points)

4. **When choosing activities to do with friends, you:**
   - A. Suggest things you genuinely enjoy, even if they're different. (3 points)
   - B. Go along with whatever the group wants. (1 point)

- o   C. Pretend to enjoy whatever everyone else likes. (0 points)

5. **How do you handle feedback from others?**
   - o   A. Accept it openly and reflect on how you can improve. (3 points)
   - o   B. Listen but don't take it to heart. (1 point)
   - o   C. Get defensive and dismiss it. (0 points)

6. **When you're feeling down, you:**
   - o   A. Share your feelings with a close friend or family member. (3 points)
   - o   B. Keep it to yourself and put on a brave face. (1 point)
   - o   C. Pretend everything is fine and hide your emotions. (0 points)

7. **If you disagree with a friend's decision, you:**
   - o   A. Share your concerns respectfully and honestly. (3 points)
   - o   B. Avoid the topic to keep the peace. (1 point)
   - o   C. Agree with them even if you have doubts. (0 points)

8. **When someone compliments you, you:**
   - o   A. Thank them and accept the compliment graciously. (3 points)
   - o   B. Downplay the compliment and shift the focus. (1 point)
   - o   C. Brush it off and change the subject. (0 points)

9. **In a new social setting, you:**
   - o   A. Be yourself and let your true personality shine. (3 points)
   - o   B. Observe others first and then decide how to act. (1 point)
   - o   C. Try to fit in by mimicking others. (0 points)

10. **When making decisions, you:**

- o   A. Follow your own values and instincts. (3 points)
  - o   B. Consider others' opinions but stay true to yourself. (1 point)
  - o   C. Rely on others to make the decision for you. (0 points)

Scoring:

- **24-30 points**: You are highly authentic and genuinely care for others. Your true self shines through in your actions!
- **16-23 points**: You show a good level of authenticity but there's room for improvement. Focus on being more true to yourself in challenging situations.
- **8-15 points**: You have some authenticity but often miss opportunities to show it. Try to be more mindful of your actions and their impact on others.
- **0-7 points**: Authenticity is not your strong suit. Consider working on understanding and valuing your true self more deeply.

Reflection: Based on your score, think about areas where you can improve your authenticity and caring behaviors. Consider practicing self-reflection, embracing vulnerability, and being honest in your interactions. Authenticity is foundational to building meaningful connections and creating a fulfilling life.

GENUINELY CARING

POWER #4 – **ALTRUISM**

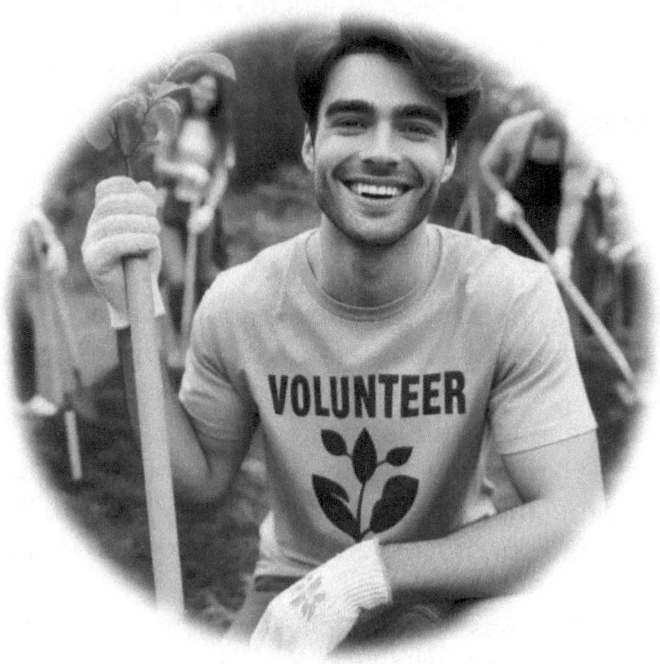

Developing altruism involves cultivating a genuine concern for the well-being of others and taking actions to benefit them, often without expecting anything in return. Here are some effective ways to develop and nurture altruism:

PRACTICE EMPATHY:

- Put Yourself in Others' Shoes: Understand and share the feelings of others, which can motivate compassionate actions.
- Listen Actively: Pay attention to others' emotions and perspectives to better understand their needs.

VOLUNTEER AND GET INVOLVED:

- Find Opportunities: Seek out local charities, community organizations, or volunteer groups where you can contribute your time and skills.
- Commit Regularly: Make volunteering a consistent part of your routine to have a sustained impact.

CULTIVATE GRATITUDE:

- Appreciate What You Have: Reflect on your own blessings and privileges, which can inspire a desire to give back to those less fortunate.
- Express Thanks: Show appreciation to others for their kindness and support, fostering a positive cycle of generosity.

EDUCATE YOURSELF:

- Learn About Social Issues: Educate yourself about issues such as poverty, homelessness, healthcare disparities, and environmental challenges.
- Stay Informed: Stay updated on current events and developments in areas where your altruistic efforts can make a difference.

SET A POSITIVE EXAMPLE:

- Be a Role Model: Demonstrate altruistic behavior in your daily life, inspiring others to do the same.
- Encourage Others: Encourage friends, family, and colleagues to join you in altruistic activities and initiatives.

PRACTICE RANDOM ACTS OF KINDNESS:

- Spread Positivity: Perform small acts of kindness, such as helping a stranger, offering compliments, or buying someone coffee.
- Be Creative: Find unique ways to brighten someone's day without expecting recognition or reward.

SUPPORT CAUSES YOU CARE ABOUT:

- Donate Wisely: Contribute financially to reputable charities and non-profit organizations aligned with your values and goals.
- Fundraise: Organize or participate in fundraising events to raise awareness and support for important causes.

BUILD MEANINGFUL RELATIONSHIPS:

- Connect with Others: Foster genuine connections with people from diverse backgrounds and circumstances.
- Show Compassion: Offer emotional support and assistance to friends, family, and acquaintances during challenging times.

REFLECT ON YOUR IMPACT:

- Evaluate Your Actions: Regularly assess how your altruistic efforts are benefiting others and consider ways to enhance your impact.
- Seek Feedback: Solicit feedback from recipients and stakeholders to improve your approach and effectiveness.

PRACTICE SELF-CARE:

- Maintain Balance: Take care of your own physical, emotional, and mental well-being to sustain your capacity for altruism.
- Set Boundaries: Establish healthy boundaries to prevent burnout and ensure long-term sustainability in your altruistic endeavors.

CELEBRATE ALTRUISM:

- Recognize Achievements: Acknowledge and celebrate the altruistic efforts and achievements of yourself and others in your community.
- Inspire Others: Share stories of altruism and compassion to inspire positive change and collective action.

By integrating these practices into your life, you can develop and strengthen your altruistic tendencies, making a meaningful and positive impact on individuals, communities, and society as a whole.

WHAT ALTRUISM STRATEGY OR STRATEGIES, SEEM MOST ATTRACTIVE TO **YOU** THAT WILL MAKE THE MOST IMPACT IN YOUR LIFE RIGHT NOW?

1.____

2.____

3.____

WHY WOULD THIS STRATEGY OR STRATEGIES MAKE THE MOST IMPACT IN YOUR LIFE RIGHT NOW?

1.____

____

WHAT **STUDIES** SHOW THE BENEFITS OF GENUINELY CARING FOR OTHERS USING ALTRUISM?

Research into altruism has demonstrated numerous benefits, both for individuals who practice altruistic behaviors and for society as a whole. Here are some key findings from studies that highlight the benefits of genuinely caring for others through altruism:

IMPROVED MENTAL HEALTH:

Reduced Stress and Anxiety: Studies have shown that individuals who engage in altruistic activities experience lower levels of stress and anxiety. Altruism promotes a sense of purpose and fulfillment, which contributes to overall psychological well-being.

Enhanced Life Satisfaction: Research indicates that altruism is positively correlated with higher levels of life satisfaction and happiness. Helping others and making a positive impact on their lives can increase one's own sense of fulfillment and contentment.

PHYSICAL HEALTH BENEFITS:

Better Physical Health: Altruism has been linked to improved physical health outcomes, including lower blood pressure and a reduced risk of cardiovascular disease. Engaging in altruistic behaviors may enhance immune function and promote longevity.

Faster Recovery: Studies suggest that individuals who are altruistic may recover more quickly from illnesses and surgery. Altruism may boost resilience and aid in coping with health challenges.

SOCIAL CONNECTION AND SUPPORT:

Stronger Social Bonds: Altruism fosters meaningful connections with others and strengthens social relationships. Building supportive networks through altruistic actions can provide emotional support and a sense of belonging.

Increased Trust: Altruistic behaviors contribute to the development of trust and cooperation within communities. Trustworthy individuals who prioritize others' well-being are valued members of social groups.

PSYCHOLOGICAL BENEFITS:

Enhanced Empathy and Compassion: Engaging in altruistic acts can cultivate empathy and compassion towards others. Altruism promotes understanding and sensitivity to the needs and emotions of others, fostering positive interpersonal relationships.

Personal Growth: Altruism encourages personal growth and self-discovery. Individuals who practice altruism often report a greater sense of self-worth and fulfillment as they contribute to the welfare of others.

COGNITIVE BENEFITS:

Improved Cognitive Function: Some research suggests that altruism may enhance cognitive function and brain health. Engaging in prosocial behaviors, such as volunteering or helping others, may stimulate neural pathways associated with reward and positive emotions.

Reduced Cognitive Decline: Altruism has been associated with a lower risk of cognitive decline and dementia in older adults. The social engagement and sense of purpose derived from altruistic activities may support cognitive resilience.

COMMUNITY AND SOCIETAL BENEFITS:

Promotion of Social Justice: Altruism plays a role in advocating for social justice and equity. Individuals who advocate for others' rights and well-being contribute to the creation of fairer and more inclusive communities.

Collective Well-Being: Altruism contributes to the overall well-being of society by addressing social challenges and promoting positive social change. Altruistic individuals and organizations are instrumental in fostering community resilience and addressing community needs.

These findings underscore the multifaceted benefits of genuinely caring for others through altruism. By practicing altruistic behaviors, individuals not only enhance their own well-being but also contribute to creating a more compassionate and supportive society.

<u>WHAT DO WE NOW KNOW</u> ABOUT GENUINELY CARING USING ALTRUISM?

ALTRUISM AND CARING QUIZ

Instructions: Answer each question honestly based on your typical behavior. At the end, tally your points to see how altruistic and caring you are!

1. **When you see someone struggling with heavy bags, you:**
   - A. Offer to help them carry their bags to their destination. (3 points)
   - B. Consider helping but decide not to get involved. (1 point)
   - C. Ignore them and continue on your way. (0 points)
2. **If a friend is going through a tough time, you:**
   - A. Reach out to them to offer support and comfort. (3 points)
   - B. Wait for them to reach out to you for help. (1 point)
   - C. Assume they'll figure it out on their own. (0 points)
3. **During a charity fundraiser, you:**
   - A. Donate money and volunteer your time to help organize the event. (3 points)
   - B. Donate a small amount of money when asked. (1 point)
   - C. Ignore the fundraiser altogether. (0 points)
4. **When you find something valuable that someone lost, you:**
   - A. Try to locate the owner and return it to them. (3 points)
   - B. Keep it for yourself or ignore it. (0 points)

- o C. Consider returning it but decide it's too much trouble. (1 point)

5. **If you witness someone being treated unfairly, you:**
   - o A. Speak up and intervene to support the person being treated unfairly. (3 points)
   - o B. Feel bad about it but don't get involved. (1 point)
   - o C. Ignore it and avoid getting into any conflicts. (0 points)

6. **When you have extra food or resources, you:**
   - o A. Share them with others who are in need. (3 points)
   - o B. Save them for later or throw them away. (0 points)
   - o C. Consider donating them but often forget or procrastinate. (1 point)

7. **How often do you volunteer your time to help others?**
   - o A. Regularly volunteer and actively seek out opportunities to help. (3 points)
   - o B. Occasionally volunteer when it's convenient. (1 point)
   - o C. Rarely or never volunteer. (0 points)

8. **If a colleague is overwhelmed with work, you:**
   - o A. Offer to help them complete their tasks or find solutions. (3 points)
   - o B. Sympathize with them but don't offer assistance. (1 point)
   - o C. Assume they should manage their workload on their own. (0 points)

9. **When interacting with strangers, you:**
   - o A. Treat them with kindness and consideration. (3 points)
   - o B. Remain neutral and polite. (1 point)
   - o C. Keep to yourself and avoid engaging with them. (0 points)

10. **If you could make a significant positive impact on someone's life by sacrificing something important to you, you would:**
   - A. Make the sacrifice to help them without hesitation. (3 points)
   - B. Consider the sacrifice but hesitate to act. (1 point)
   - C. Prioritize your own needs and interests. (0 points)

Scoring:

- **27-30 points**: You are highly altruistic and genuinely caring for others. Your actions consistently demonstrate your compassion and willingness to help those in need.
- **18-26 points**: You show a good level of altruism but there's room for improvement. Consider seeking out more opportunities to help others and making altruism a more consistent part of your life.
- **9-17 points**: You have some altruistic tendencies but often miss opportunities to demonstrate caring for others. Focus on being more proactive and compassionate in your actions.
- **0-8 points**: Altruism is not currently a priority in your life. Reflect on ways to develop a greater sense of empathy and compassion towards others.

Reflection: Based on your score, think about areas where you can enhance your altruistic behaviors. Practicing empathy, actively seeking opportunities to help others, and making a positive impact in your community can contribute to a more fulfilling and compassionate life. Every small act of kindness counts towards creating a more caring and supportive world!

POWER #5 – **RELIABILITY**

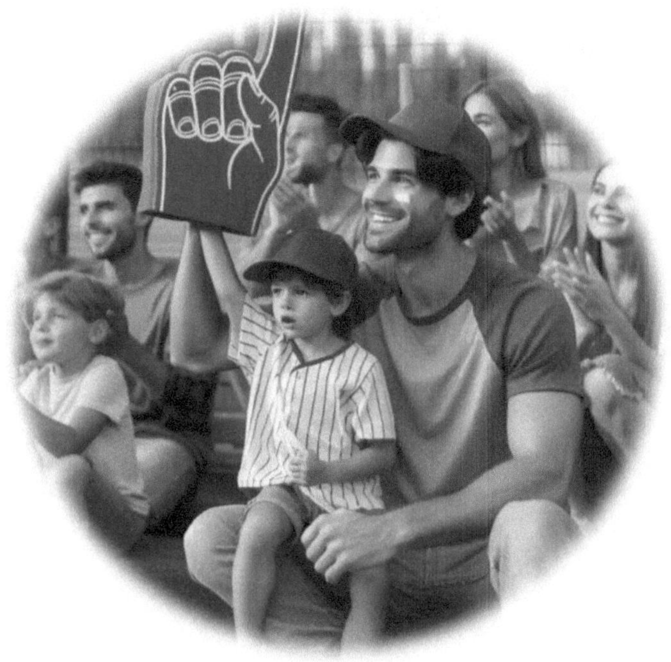

Developing reliability involves establishing a reputation for consistently delivering on commitments and being trustworthy in various contexts. Here are some effective ways to cultivate and enhance reliability:

SET CLEAR EXPECTATIONS:

- Communicate Clearly: Ensure that you understand expectations clearly and ask questions if anything is unclear.
- Clarify Deadlines and Requirements: Confirm timelines, deliverables, and any specific requirements upfront.

PRIORITIZE ORGANIZATION AND TIME MANAGEMENT:

- Use Tools and Systems: Utilize calendars, task lists, or project management software to stay organized.
- Allocate Sufficient Time: Plan ahead and allocate adequate time for each task or commitment to avoid rushing or missing deadlines.

HONOR COMMITMENTS CONSISTENTLY:

- Meet Deadlines: Deliver work or fulfill promises on time or even ahead of schedule whenever possible.
- Follow Through: Complete tasks thoroughly and with attention to detail, meeting agreed-upon quality standards.

COMMUNICATE EFFECTIVELY:

- Provide Updates: Keep stakeholders informed of progress, setbacks, or changes in plans promptly and transparently.
- Be Responsive: Respond to messages, emails, or inquiries in a timely manner, demonstrating reliability in communication.

BUILD TRUST THROUGH DEPENDABILITY:

- Be Predictable: Consistently demonstrate reliability in both routine and challenging situations.
- Handle Responsibilities: Take ownership of your responsibilities and demonstrate accountability for your actions.

LEARN FROM FEEDBACK:

- Seek Feedback: Request constructive feedback from colleagues, supervisors, or clients to identify areas for improvement.
- Adapt and Improve: Act on feedback to refine your approach and enhance your reliability over time.

STAY FOCUSED AND AVOID OVERCOMMITTING:

- Prioritize Tasks: Focus on completing tasks in order of importance to prevent feeling overwhelmed.
- Manage Workload: Avoid taking on too many commitments simultaneously to maintain high-quality work and reliability.

CULTIVATE SELF-DISCIPLINE AND ACCOUNTABILITY:

- Set Goals: Establish realistic goals and milestones to track progress and maintain motivation.
- Hold Yourself Accountable: Take responsibility for your actions and commitments, demonstrating integrity and reliability.

BE PROACTIVE AND ANTICIPATE NEEDS:

- Plan Ahead: Anticipate potential challenges or obstacles and develop contingency plans to mitigate risks.
- Offer Support: Extend assistance to others when needed, demonstrating reliability in supporting team or community efforts.

REFLECT AND IMPROVE CONTINUOUSLY:

- Evaluate Performance: Regularly assess your reliability in meeting commitments and achieving goals.
- Commit to Growth: Continuously seek opportunities to learn, grow, and refine your skills in reliability.

By focusing on these strategies, you can develop a reputation for reliability both personally and professionally, fostering trust and confidence in your abilities to consistently deliver on your promises and obligations.

WHAT RELIABILITY STRATEGY OR STRATEGIES, SEEM MOST ATTRACTIVE TO **YOU** THAT WILL MAKE THE MOST IMPACT IN YOUR LIFE RIGHT NOW?

1.__________________________________

2.__________________________________

3.__________________________________

WHY WOULD THIS STRATEGY OR STRATEGIES MAKE THE MOST IMPACT IN YOUR LIFE RIGHT NOW?

1.__________________________________

____

WHAT **STUDIES** SHOW THE BENEFITS OF GENUINELY CARING FOR OTHERS USING RELIABILITY?

Research specifically highlighting the benefits of reliability in the context of genuinely caring for others is somewhat limited, but there are numerous studies that explore the broader impact of reliability on relationships, mental health, workplace dynamics, and social cohesion. Here are some key findings that illustrate the benefits of being reliable and how it translates into genuinely caring for others:

TRUST AND RELATIONSHIP QUALITY:

Building Trust: Reliability is foundational in building and maintaining trust in relationships. A study published in the *Journal of Personality and Social Psychology* found that consistent, reliable behavior fosters trust and strengthens interpersonal bonds.

Relationship Satisfaction: Research indicates that reliability contributes to higher satisfaction in romantic relationships. Partners who perceive each other as reliable are more likely to experience stability and satisfaction.

MENTAL HEALTH AND WELL-BEING:

Reduced Anxiety and Stress: A study in the *Journal of Health and Social Behavior* found that reliable social support can significantly reduce anxiety and stress levels. Knowing that others are dependable provides a sense of security and emotional comfort.

Increased Psychological Well-Being: Reliable relationships are linked to higher levels of psychological well-being. The assurance that others will fulfill their commitments enhances overall life satisfaction and happiness.

WORKPLACE PERFORMANCE:

Employee Productivity: In organizational settings, reliability is associated with improved job performance and productivity. A study in the *Academy of Management Journal* showed that reliable employees contribute to more efficient and effective team dynamics, leading to better overall organizational performance.

Job Satisfaction: Research in the *Journal of Applied Psychology* highlights that employees who work in reliable environments report higher job satisfaction and morale. Reliability in leadership and peer support fosters a positive and motivating work culture.

SOCIAL SUPPORT AND COMMUNITY COHESION:

Strengthening Social Networks: A study in the *American Journal of Community Psychology* found that reliability within social networks strengthens community ties and enhances social cohesion. Communities where members can rely on each other are more resilient and supportive.

Reduced Loneliness: Reliable relationships reduce feelings of loneliness and isolation. Research published in *Social Science & Medicine* indicates that individuals with dependable social connections have lower rates of loneliness and better mental health outcomes.

CONFLICT RESOLUTION AND HARMONY:

Effective Conflict Resolution: Reliable individuals are better at resolving conflicts constructively. A study in the *Journal of Conflict Resolution* found that reliability in communication and behavior fosters mutual respect and effective problem-solving.

Enhanced Social Harmony: Consistency and reliability in behavior contribute to social harmony by reducing misunderstandings and fostering a cooperative environment.

These findings collectively suggest that reliability plays a crucial role in fostering trust, mental health, workplace satisfaction, social cohesion, and effective conflict resolution. By being reliable, individuals demonstrate genuine care and support for others, leading to numerous positive outcomes in both personal and professional contexts.

<u>**WHAT DO WE NOW KNOW**</u> ABOUT GENUINELY CARING USING RELIABILITY?

RELIABILITY AND CARING QUIZ

Instructions: Answer each question honestly based on your typical behavior. At the end, tally your points to see how reliable and caring you are!

1. **When you promise to meet a friend at a specific time, you:**
   - A. Always arrive on time or even a few minutes early. (3 points)
   - B. Sometimes arrive late due to unforeseen circumstances. (1 point)
   - C. Frequently arrive late or cancel plans last minute. (0 points)

2. **If someone asks for your help with a task, you:**
   - A. Prioritize their request and follow through promptly. (3 points)
   - B. Consider helping but may forget or delay in assisting. (1 point)
   - C. Often decline or avoid helping altogether. (0 points)

3. **When given a work assignment with a deadline, you:**
   - A. Complete it ahead of schedule or by the deadline without fail. (3 points)
   - B. Finish it on time most of the time, but occasionally miss deadlines. (1 point)
   - C. Frequently miss deadlines or submit incomplete work. (0 points)

4. **If you agree to keep a secret for a friend, you:**
   - A. Honor their trust and keep the secret confidential. (3 points)
   - B. Struggle to keep the secret and may inadvertently share it. (1 point)

- C. Have difficulty keeping secrets and often share them with others. (0 points)

5. **In group projects or team settings, you are known for:**
    - A. Taking responsibility for your part and ensuring tasks are completed on time. (3 points)
    - B. Contributing to the team effort but sometimes rely on others to finish tasks. (1 point)
    - C. Depending on others to do most of the work or not contributing significantly. (0 points)

6. **When you commit to attending social events or gatherings, you:**
    - A. Attend as planned unless circumstances prevent you from doing so. (3 points)
    - B. Occasionally cancel plans due to other priorities or changes in schedule. (1 point)
    - C. Frequently cancel plans last minute or simply don't show up. (0 points)

7. **If you borrow something from a friend, you make sure to:**
    - A. Return it promptly and in the same condition or better. (3 points)
    - B. Return it eventually but may forget or take longer than expected. (1 point)
    - C. Often forget to return borrowed items or return them damaged. (0 points)

8. **When asked to assist with a community project or volunteer effort, you:**
    - A. Commit to helping and follow through with your contributions. (3 points)
    - B. Consider participating but may not always follow through due to other commitments. (1 point)

- o C. Rarely or never participate in community or volunteer activities. (0 points)

9. **If you make a mistake, you are known for:**
   - o A. Acknowledging the mistake and taking steps to correct it. (3 points)
   - o B. Sometimes admitting fault but may avoid addressing it fully. (1 point)
   - o C. Blaming others or denying responsibility for mistakes. (0 points)

10. **When offering support to friends or family in need, you:**
    - o A. Consistently provide reliable support and follow through with your offers. (3 points)
    - o B. Offer support when convenient but may not always follow through consistently. (1 point)
    - o C. Often make promises of support but fail to deliver when needed. (0 points)

Scoring:

- **27-30 points**: You are highly reliable and genuinely caring for others. Your consistency and dependability make you a valuable friend and team member!
- **18-26 points**: You demonstrate good reliability but there's room for improvement. Focus on being more consistent in fulfilling commitments and supporting others.
- **9-17 points**: You have some reliability but often miss opportunities to demonstrate caring for others through your actions. Consider becoming more proactive and dependable.
- **0-8 points**: Reliability is not currently a strong suit. Reflect on ways to develop a greater sense

of responsibility and follow-through in your interactions with others.

Reflection: Based on your score, think about areas where you can enhance your reliability and caring behaviors. Practice setting and meeting expectations, communicating clearly, and prioritizing commitments to build trust and strengthen your relationships. Being reliable is key to demonstrating genuine care and support for others!

GENUINELY CARING

POWER #6 – **SUPPORTIVENESS**

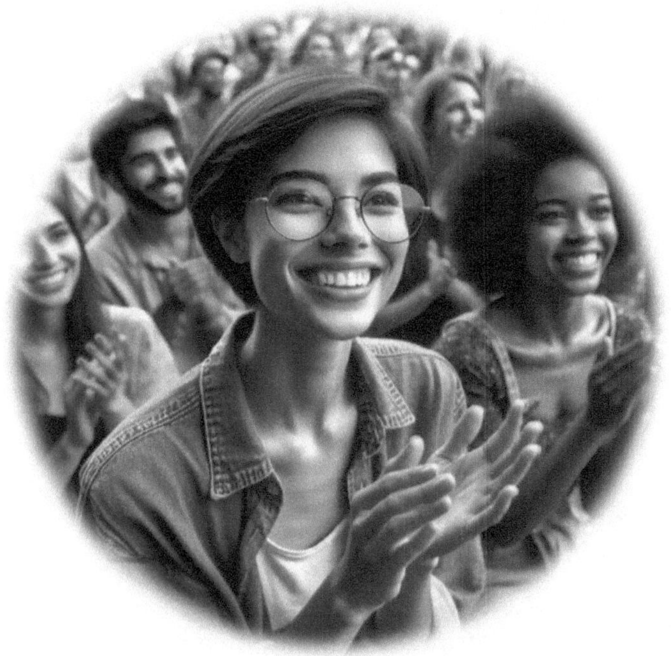

Developing supportiveness involves cultivating a mindset and behaviors that prioritize the well-being and success of others. Here are some effective ways to develop and enhance supportiveness:

ACTIVE LISTENING:

- Pay Attention: Listen attentively to others without interrupting or planning your response.
- Show Empathy: Understand others' perspectives and emotions, validating their feelings and experiences.

OFFER EMOTIONAL SUPPORT:

- Be Present: Provide reassurance and comfort to others during challenging times.
- Validate Feelings: Acknowledge and respect their emotions, even if you don't fully understand their situation.

PROVIDE PRACTICAL HELP:

- Offer Assistance: Be proactive in offering tangible help, such as helping with tasks or running errands.
- Ask How You Can Help: Offer specific ways to assist based on their needs and preferences.

CELEBRATE ACHIEVEMENTS:

- Acknowledge Successes: Celebrate others' accomplishments and milestones, showing genuine happiness for their achievements.
- Encourage Growth: Support their ambitions and efforts to grow professionally and personally.

BE RELIABLE AND DEPENDABLE:

- Follow Through: Honor commitments and promises, demonstrating consistency and reliability.
- Offer Consistent Support: Be there consistently, especially during difficult times or when support is needed.

PROVIDE CONSTRUCTIVE FEEDBACK:

- Offer Guidance: Provide feedback in a constructive and supportive manner to help others improve.

- Focus on Improvement: Offer suggestions for growth and development rather than criticism.

ENCOURAGE AND MOTIVATE:

- Provide Encouragement: Offer words of encouragement and motivation to inspire others during challenges.
- Be Positive: Maintain a positive attitude and outlook, especially when supporting others through tough situations.

CREATE A SUPPORTIVE ENVIRONMENT:

- Foster Inclusivity: Create an environment where everyone feels valued and included.
- Promote Collaboration: Encourage teamwork and collaboration to achieve common goals and objectives.

SHOW RESPECT AND CONSIDERATION:

- Respect Boundaries: Respect others' boundaries and preferences when offering support.
- Be Considerate: Consider their feelings, preferences, and needs when providing assistance or guidance.

LEAD BY EXAMPLE:

- Demonstrate Supportiveness: Model supportive behaviors in your interactions with others.
- Inspire Others: Encourage others to be supportive and create a culture of supportiveness in your community or workplace.

REFLECT AND IMPROVE:

- Seek Feedback: Ask for feedback on how you can be more supportive and responsive to others' needs.
- Continuous Learning: Learn from experiences and adjust your approach to better meet the needs of those you support.

By focusing on these strategies, you can cultivate a supportive mindset and behaviors that contribute to building strong, trusting relationships and fostering a positive, collaborative environment where everyone feels valued and encouraged.

WHAT SUPPORTIVENESS STRATEGY OR STRATEGIES
SEEM MOST ATTRACTIVE TO **YOU** THAT WILL MAKE
THE MOST IMPACT IN YOUR LIFE RIGHT NOW?

1.____

2.____

3.____

WHY WOULD THIS STRATEGY OR STRATEGIES MAKE
THE MOST IMPACT IN YOUR LIFE RIGHT NOW?

1____

____

WHAT **STUDIES** SHOW THE BENEFITS OF GENUINELY CARING FOR OTHERS USING SUPPORTIVENESS?

Research on supportiveness highlights numerous benefits for both the giver and the receiver in various contexts, such as mental health, relationships, workplace environments, and community well-being. Here are some key studies and findings that demonstrate the benefits of genuinely caring for others using supportiveness:

MENTAL HEALTH AND WELL-BEING:

Reduction in Stress and Anxiety: A study published in the *Journal of Health and Social Behavior* found that individuals who receive social support experience lower levels of stress and anxiety. Emotional support from friends and family helps buffer the negative effects of stress.

Improved Psychological Well-Being: Research published in *Psychological Science* indicates that providing and receiving support is linked to higher levels of happiness and life satisfaction. Supportive interactions enhance overall psychological well-being.

RELATIONSHIP QUALITY:

Increased Relationship Satisfaction: A study in the *Journal of Personality and Social Psychology* found that supportive behaviors, such as providing emotional and practical assistance, contribute to greater relationship satisfaction and stability.

Enhanced Communication: Supportive interactions improve communication between partners, leading to more effective conflict resolution and deeper emotional connections, as reported in research published in the *Journal of Social and Personal Relationships*.

PHYSICAL HEALTH:

Better Immune Function: Research in *Psychosomatic Medicine* suggests that social support can enhance immune function, making individuals more resilient to illnesses. Emotional support helps reduce the physiological impact of stress.

Reduced Risk of Chronic Illness: A study in the *American Journal of Epidemiology* found that strong social support networks are associated with a lower risk of chronic illnesses such as cardiovascular disease. Supportive behaviors promote healthier lifestyles and adherence to medical advice.

RESILIENCE AND COPING:

Enhanced Coping Mechanisms: Individuals who receive and provide support are better equipped to handle life's challenges and adversities. A study published in *Health Psychology* found that social support improves coping strategies and resilience.

Recovery from Trauma: Research in the *Journal of Traumatic Stress* highlights the critical role of supportive social networks in recovery from traumatic experiences. Emotional and practical support facilitate healing and adaptation.

WORKPLACE OUTCOMES:

Higher Job Satisfaction: Supportive work environments are linked to higher job satisfaction and employee morale, as demonstrated in a study published in the *Journal of Occupational Health Psychology*.

Improved Performance and Productivity: Research in the *Journal of Applied Psychology* indicates that employees who feel supported by their peers and supervisors tend to perform better and are more productive. Supportive behaviors enhance motivation, engagement, and commitment to organizational goals.

COMMUNITY AND SOCIAL BENEFITS:

Increased Community Cohesion: Supportive communities, where members help each other, show stronger social bonds and a greater sense of belonging. This was demonstrated in a study published in the *American Journal of Community Psychology*.

Reduction in Social Isolation: Supportive behaviors help reduce feelings of loneliness and social isolation, particularly among vulnerable populations. Research published in *Social Science & Medicine* indicates that social support networks provide a sense of connection and purpose.

These studies collectively highlight the multifaceted benefits of supportiveness, demonstrating its critical role in enhancing mental and physical health, relationship quality, workplace satisfaction, and community well-being. By genuinely caring for others through supportive behaviors, individuals and communities can experience a wide range of positive outcomes that contribute to overall quality of life.

<u>WHAT DO WE NOW KNOW</u> ABOUT GENUINELY CARING USING SUPPORTIVENESS?

HOW SUPPORTIVE ARE YOU? QUIZ

Instructions: Answer each question honestly based on your typical behavior. At the end, tally your points to see how supportive you are!

1. **A friend calls you late at night, feeling upset. You:**
   - o   A. Answer the call and listen to them, offering comfort and support. (3 points)
   - o   B. Answer but keep the conversation short, as you're tired. (2 points)
   - o   C. Let it go to voicemail and plan to call back the next day. (1 point)
2. **Your colleague is struggling with a project. You:**
   - o   A. Offer to help them and spend extra time to ensure they succeed. (3 points)
   - o   B. Give them some advice but let them handle the rest. (2 points)
   - o   C. Suggest they ask someone else who might have more time. (1 point)
3. **A family member is sick and needs assistance with daily tasks. You:**
   - o   A. Rearrange your schedule to help them as much as possible. (3 points)
   - o   B. Help when you can but keep most of your plans. (2 points)
   - o   C. Check in on them occasionally but continue with your routine. (1 point)
4. **Your friend is having a bad day and shares their troubles with you. You:**

- A. Listen attentively, validate their feelings, and offer encouragement. (3 points)
- B. Listen and try to cheer them up with a joke or distraction. (2 points)
- C. Listen briefly and then suggest they focus on the positive. (1 point)

5. **In a group project, you notice someone is overwhelmed. You:**
   - A. Volunteer to take on some of their tasks to lighten their load. (3 points)
   - B. Offer to help with specific parts if they ask for it. (2 points)
   - C. Encourage them to manage their time better. (1 point)

6. **Your neighbor is having car trouble and needs a ride to work. You:**
   - A. Offer to drive them to work and back until their car is fixed. (3 points)
   - B. Offer to drive them for a couple of days until they find another solution. (2 points)
   - C. Suggest they take public transportation or find another ride. (1 point)

7. **A friend is excited about a new hobby and wants to share it with you. You:**
   - A. Show genuine interest and even participate with them occasionally. (3 points)
   - B. Listen and ask a few questions but don't show much enthusiasm. (2 points)
   - C. Acknowledge it briefly and then change the subject. (1 point)

8. **A coworker asks for your feedback on their work. You:**

- o   A. Provide detailed, constructive feedback and offer to help with improvements. (3 points)
- o   B. Give some general feedback and encourage them to keep working on it. (2 points)
- o   C. Offer brief, vague feedback and suggest they seek a second opinion. (1 point)

9. **A friend is moving and needs help packing. You:**
- o   A. Spend a whole day helping them pack and organize their belongings. (3 points)
- o   B. Help for a couple of hours and then move on to your own plans. (2 points)
- o   C. Lend them some packing supplies and wish them luck. (1 point)

10. **Your partner has an important event coming up and is feeling nervous. You:**
- o   A. Offer constant reassurance and help them prepare thoroughly. (3 points)
- o   B. Reassure them and help with some preparations. (2 points)
- o   C. Tell them they'll do great and leave them to prepare on their own. (1 point)

Scoring:

- **25-30 points**: You are highly supportive and genuinely care for others. Your friends, family, and colleagues can always count on you for emotional and practical support!
- **18-24 points**: You are generally supportive but have room for improvement. Focus on being more proactive and consistent in offering help and encouragement.

- **10-17 points**: You show some supportiveness, but often miss opportunities to be there for others. Consider making more of an effort to offer your assistance and listen actively.
- **0-9 points**: Supportiveness is not currently a strong suit. Reflect on ways to be more present and helpful in the lives of those around you.

Reflection: Based on your score, think about areas where you can enhance your supportiveness. Practice active listening, offer help proactively, and be consistent in your supportive behaviors. Being genuinely caring and supportive can strengthen your relationships and contribute positively to the well-being of those around you!

GENUINELY CARING

POWER #7 – **HUMILITY**

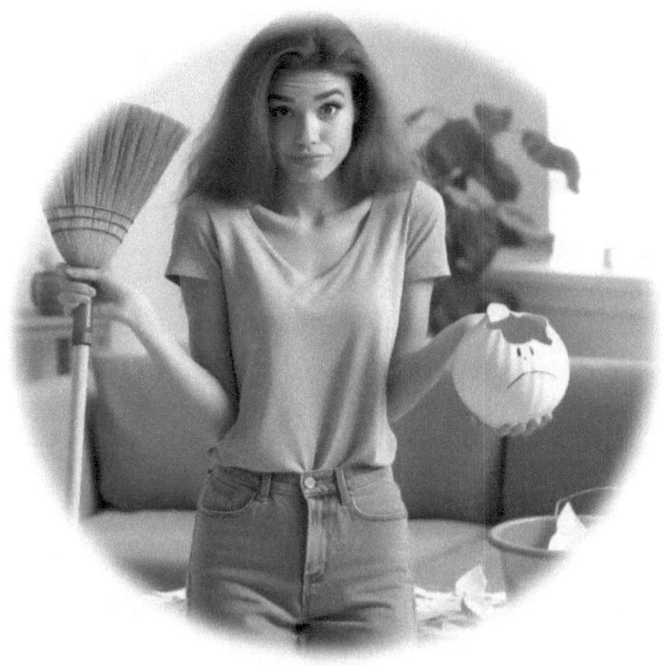

Developing humility involves cultivating a mindset that values others, acknowledges one's limitations, and maintains a balanced sense of self-worth. Here are some effective ways to develop and enhance humility:

SELF-REFLECTION:

- Regularly Reflect on Your Actions: Take time to reflect on your behavior, decisions, and interactions. Consider what went well and what could have been handled better.
- Acknowledge Your Mistakes: Be honest about your mistakes and take responsibility for them. Learn from these experiences to improve yourself.

116

PRACTICE GRATITUDE:

- Appreciate What You Have: Regularly acknowledge the positive aspects of your life and express gratitude for them. This helps you stay grounded and aware of the contributions of others to your success.
- Thank Others: Show appreciation for the help and support you receive from others. Acknowledge their efforts and express sincere thanks.

SEEK FEEDBACK:

- Ask for Constructive Criticism: Invite feedback from trusted friends, colleagues, or mentors. Be open to their suggestions and use them to improve yourself.
- Listen Actively: Pay attention to what others say without becoming defensive. Consider their perspectives and apply their advice where applicable.

SERVE OTHERS:

- Volunteer Your Time: Engage in activities that help others without expecting anything in return. Volunteering can broaden your perspective and reinforce the importance of selflessness.
- Support Your Community: Get involved in community projects or support causes that are meaningful to you. Contributing to the well-being of others fosters a sense of humility.

LEARN CONTINUOUSLY:

- Pursue Knowledge: Stay curious and open to learning new things. Recognize that there is always more to learn and that you can benefit from the knowledge and experiences of others.

- Embrace Lifelong Learning: Take courses, read books, and engage in activities that expand your understanding and skills. Humility grows when you acknowledge that you don't know everything.

CULTIVATE EMPATHY:

- Understand Others' Perspectives: Make an effort to see situations from others' viewpoints. Empathy fosters respect and appreciation for the experiences and challenges of others.
- Show Compassion: Respond to others with kindness and understanding. Support them in their struggles and celebrate their successes.

BE MINDFUL:

- Practice Mindfulness: Engage in mindfulness exercises, such as meditation or deep breathing, to stay present and aware of your thoughts and actions.
- Stay Grounded: Mindfulness helps you maintain a balanced perspective, reducing ego-driven thoughts and behaviors.

AVOID COMPARISONS:

- Focus on Your Own Journey: Avoid comparing yourself to others. Recognize that everyone has their own unique path and challenges.
- Celebrate Others' Successes: Be genuinely happy for the achievements of others without feeling threatened or envious.

CULTIVATE A SENSE OF HUMOR:

- Laugh at Yourself: Don't take yourself too seriously. Being able to laugh at your own mistakes and shortcomings is a sign of humility.
- Enjoy Life's Simple Pleasures: Find joy in everyday moments and appreciate the small things in life.

MODEL HUMILITY:

- Lead by Example: Demonstrate humility in your actions and interactions with others. Show respect, kindness, and openness in all situations.
- Inspire Others: Encourage those around you to adopt humble behaviors by exemplifying these traits in your own life.

By incorporating these practices into your daily life, you can develop and enhance your sense of humility. This, in turn, can lead to more meaningful relationships, personal growth, and a deeper understanding of yourself and others.

WHAT HUMILITY STRATEGY OR STRATEGIES, SEEM MOST ATTRACTIVE TO **YOU** THAT WILL MAKE THE MOST IMPACT IN YOUR LIFE RIGHT NOW?

1.____

2.____

3.____

WHY WOULD THIS STRATEGY OR STRATEGIES MAKE THE MOST IMPACT IN YOUR LIFE RIGHT NOW?

1.____

____

WHAT **STUDIES** SHOW THE BENEFITS OF GENUINELY CARING FOR OTHERS USING HUMILITY?

Studies on humility and its effects often highlight the benefits of genuinely caring for others through humble behavior. Humility is associated with various positive outcomes in personal relationships, mental health, and leadership effectiveness. Here are some key findings from research that illustrate the benefits of practicing humility in the context of caring for others:

IMPROVED RELATIONSHIPS:

Relationship Satisfaction: A study published in the *Journal of Positive Psychology* found that humility in romantic relationships is linked to higher levels of satisfaction and commitment. Humble partners are more willing to admit mistakes, forgive, and show empathy, which strengthens the relationship.

Greater Social Bonds: Research in *Personality and Individual Differences* indicated that humility enhances social bonds. People who exhibit humility are more likely to be perceived as kind, trustworthy, and likable, which fosters stronger connections with others.

MENTAL HEALTH BENEFITS:

Reduced Anxiety and Depression: A study in the *Journal of Psychology and Theology* found that humility is negatively correlated with anxiety and depression. Humility helps individuals maintain a balanced perspective on their strengths and weaknesses, reducing the pressure to be perfect and thereby lowering stress levels.

Increased Psychological Well-Being: Research published in the *Journal of Personality and Social Psychology* suggests that humility contributes to greater psychological well-being. Humble individuals tend to have a more accurate self-assessment and are less likely to experience negative emotions like pride and arrogance.

LEADERSHIP EFFECTIVENESS:

Effective Leadership: A study in the *Academy of Management Journal* found that humble leaders are more effective because they foster an inclusive environment where team members feel valued and empowered. Humble leaders are also more likely to seek input from others and make decisions that benefit the group.

Employee Satisfaction: Research in the *Journal of Management* showed that employees who perceive their leaders as humble report higher job satisfaction and engagement. Humble leaders are seen as approachable and supportive, which enhances workplace morale.

CONFLICT RESOLUTION:

Better Conflict Management: A study published in *Negotiation and Conflict Management Research* found that humility improves conflict resolution skills. Humble individuals are more likely to listen to others, acknowledge their own faults, and seek mutually beneficial solutions, leading to more effective conflict management.

COMMUNITY AND SOCIAL IMPACT:

Increased Prosocial Behavior: Research in the *Journal of Personality* indicated that humility is associated with higher levels of prosocial behavior, such as volunteering and helping others. Humble individuals are more likely to engage in acts of kindness and support their community.

Stronger Community Bonds: A study in *Psychological Science* found that communities with higher levels of humility experience stronger social cohesion and cooperation. Humility promotes an environment where individuals prioritize the collective good over personal gain.

ACADEMIC AND PERSONAL GROWTH:

Enhanced Learning and Growth: Research published in the *Journal of Educational Psychology* suggests that humility is linked to a growth mindset. Humble individuals are more open to feedback and continuous learning, which contributes to personal and academic development.

Better Academic Performance: A study in *Personality and Individual Differences* found that students who exhibit humility tend to perform better academically. Their willingness to acknowledge their limitations and seek help when needed leads to improved learning outcomes.

These studies collectively highlight the benefits of humility in various aspects of life. By genuinely caring for others through humble behavior, individuals can foster stronger relationships, enhance their mental health, become more effective leaders, and contribute positively to their communities.

<u>WHAT DO WE NOW KNOW</u> ABOUT GENUINELY CARING USING HUMILITY?

HOW HUMBLE ARE YOU IN CARING FOR OTHERS? QUIZ

Instructions: Answer each question honestly based on your typical behavior. At the end, tally your points to see how humility influences your care for others!

1. **A friend achieves something significant. You:**
   - A. Celebrate their success genuinely and ask them to share their experience. (3 points)
   - B. Congratulate them and share a similar experience of your own. (2 points)
   - C. Offer a quick congratulations and change the subject. (1 point)
2. **You made a mistake in a group project. You:**
   - A. Admit your mistake openly and suggest ways to fix it. (3 points)
   - B. Admit the mistake but downplay its impact. (2 points)
   - C. Hope no one notices and move on. (1 point)
3. **A colleague offers constructive criticism. You:**
   - A. Thank them and ask for more details to improve. (3 points)
   - B. Acknowledge it but don't engage much further. (2 points)
   - C. Get defensive and justify your actions. (1 point)
4. **During a team discussion, you:**
   - A. Listen attentively to others' ideas and build on them. (3 points)
   - B. Share your ideas and listen when you're interested. (2 points)

- C. Focus mainly on getting your own ideas across. (1 point)

5. **You're recognized for an achievement. You:**
   - A. Share the credit with everyone who helped you. (3 points)
   - B. Accept the recognition but don't mention others' contributions. (2 points)
   - C. Take all the credit for yourself. (1 point)

6. **A friend needs help with a task you're good at. You:**
   - A. Offer to help and patiently teach them. (3 points)
   - B. Help them quickly without much explanation. (2 points)
   - C. Suggest they figure it out themselves. (1 point)

7. **Someone disagrees with your opinion. You:**
   - A. Listen to their perspective and consider it thoughtfully. (3 points)
   - B. Acknowledge their view but stick to your own opinion. (2 points)
   - C. Argue your point and dismiss their perspective. (1 point)

8. **You're leading a group project. You:**
   - A. Encourage everyone to contribute ideas and collaborate. (3 points)
   - B. Lead the project but make most of the decisions yourself. (2 points)
   - C. Take control and direct everyone's tasks. (1 point)

9. **A friend shares a personal struggle. You:**
   - A. Listen empathetically and offer your support without judgment. (3 points)
   - B. Offer advice based on your own experiences. (2 points)
   - C. Give a quick response and suggest they move on. (1 point)

10. **You receive an award. You:**
  - o   A. Express gratitude and highlight the help you received from others. (3 points)
  - o   B. Accept it graciously but focus on your own efforts. (2 points)
  - o   C. Accept it proudly, focusing on your achievements. (1 point)

Scoring:

- **25-30 points**: You have a high level of humility and genuinely care for others. Your humble attitude fosters strong, supportive relationships and makes you a valued friend and colleague.
- **18-24 points**: You show humility but have room for improvement. Focus on listening more, sharing credit, and being open to others' perspectives.
- **10-17 points**: Your humility is somewhat lacking. Reflect on how you can be more humble in your interactions and genuinely care for others.
- **0-9 points**: Humility is not a strong suit for you. Consider the benefits of humility and how adopting a more humble attitude can improve your relationships and personal growth.

Reflection: Based on your score, think about areas where you can enhance your humility. Practice active listening, acknowledge others' contributions, and be open to feedback. Humility can strengthen your relationships and lead to a more fulfilling and supportive life.

GENUINELY CARING

POWER #8 – PATIENCE

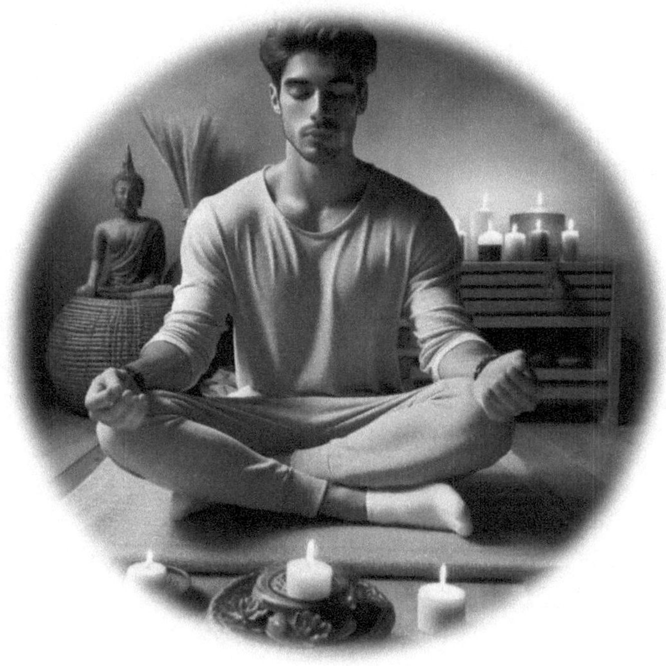

Developing patience can be challenging, but it's a valuable skill that can improve many aspects of life. Here are some of the best ways to cultivate patience:

MINDFULNESS AND MEDITATION

- Practice Mindfulness: Pay attention to the present moment without judgment. This can help you become more aware of your reactions and develop a calmer mindset.
- Meditate Regularly: Meditation helps to train your mind to stay calm and focused, which can increase your patience.

DEEP BREATHING EXERCISES

- Breathing Techniques: When you feel impatient, take deep, slow breaths. This can help calm your mind and body, making it easier to respond with patience.

SET REALISTIC EXPECTATIONS

- Manage Expectations: Understand that things often take time. Set realistic goals and timeframes to avoid unnecessary frustration.

PRACTICE GRATITUDE

- Gratitude Journaling: Keep a journal to regularly note things you are grateful for. This shift in focus can help you become more patient by appreciating what you have.

DEVELOP EMPATHY

- Put Yourself in Others' Shoes: Try to understand situations from other people's perspectives. This can help you be more patient in interactions and reduce frustration.

BREAK TASKS INTO SMALLER STEPS

- Incremental Progress: Breaking tasks into smaller, manageable steps can make them feel less overwhelming and reduce impatience.

REGULAR PHYSICAL ACTIVITY

- Exercise: Physical activity can help reduce stress and improve your mood, making it easier to stay patient.

CULTIVATE A GROWTH MINDSET

- Embrace Challenges: View challenges as opportunities to learn and grow rather than as obstacles. This mindset can help you develop patience through perseverance.

PRACTICE DELAYED GRATIFICATION

- Wait for Rewards: Intentionally delay rewards or satisfaction to train yourself to wait. This can strengthen your patience over time.

STAY POSITIVE

- Positive Self-Talk: Encourage yourself with positive affirmations and remind yourself that patience will benefit you in the long run.

ENGAGE IN HOBBIES

- Pursue Patience-Building Activities: Hobbies like gardening, knitting, or puzzles require time and attention, helping you build patience naturally.

SEEK SUPPORT

- Talk to Others: Discussing your challenges with friends, family, or a therapist can provide new perspectives and support in developing patience.

Developing patience is a gradual process that requires consistent effort. By incorporating these strategies into your daily life, you can become more patient and improve your overall well-being.

WHAT PATIENCE STRATEGY OR STRATEGIES, SEEM MOST ATTRACTIVE TO **YOU** THAT WILL MAKE THE MOST IMPACT IN YOUR LIFE RIGHT NOW?

1.____

2.____

3.____

WHY WOULD THIS STRATEGY OR STRATEGIES MAKE THE MOST IMPACT IN YOUR LIFE RIGHT NOW?

1.____

____

WHAT **STUDIES** SHOW THE BENEFITS OF GENUINELY CARING FOR OTHERS USING PATIENCE?

Numerous studies highlight the benefits of genuinely caring about others and how patience can enhance these benefits. Here are a few key studies:

THE ROLE OF EMPATHY AND PATIENCE IN SOCIAL RELATIONSHIPS

Study: A study published in the *Journal of Personality and Social Psychology* examined the role of empathy in social relationships.

Findings: The researchers found that individuals who exhibited high levels of empathy and patience were more likely to form stronger, more positive relationships. These individuals were better at understanding others' perspectives and managing conflicts, leading to more harmonious interactions.

PATIENCE AND WELL-BEING

Study: A study published in the *Journal of Positive Psychology* explored the relationship between patience and well-being.

Findings: The study found that individuals who practiced patience experienced higher levels of life satisfaction, reduced stress, and improved mental health. Patience allowed individuals to better cope with challenges and setbacks, enhancing their overall well-being and ability to care for others.

ALTRUISM AND PATIENCE

- Study: Research published in the *Journal of Experimental Social Psychology* investigated the link between altruism and patience.
- Findings: The study showed that individuals who displayed patience were more likely to engage in altruistic behaviors, such as helping others and volunteering. This connection suggests that patience can foster a genuine concern for others' well-being and increase pro-social behavior.

MINDFULNESS, PATIENCE, AND COMPASSION

- Study: A study in the *Mindfulness* journal examined the effects of mindfulness training on patience and compassion.
- Findings: Participants who underwent mindfulness training reported increased levels of patience and compassion. These traits were linked to improved interpersonal relationships and a greater ability to care for others without feeling overwhelmed.

PATIENCE IN LEADERSHIP

- Study: Research published in the *Leadership Quarterly* analyzed the impact of patience on leadership effectiveness.
- Findings: Leaders who demonstrated patience were found to be more effective in guiding their teams, resolving conflicts, and fostering a positive work environment. This ability to patiently support and understand team members led to higher levels of trust and collaboration.

NEUROSCIENCE OF PATIENCE AND EMPATHY

Study: A study published in *Social Cognitive and Affective Neuroscience* explored the neural basis of patience and empathy.

Findings: The research revealed that practicing patience activates brain regions associated with empathy and emotional regulation. This neural activity supports the development of caring behaviors and enhances the capacity to understand and respond to others' needs.

These studies collectively suggest that patience plays a crucial role in fostering genuine care for others. By enhancing empathy, reducing stress, promoting altruism, and improving interpersonal relationships, patience can significantly benefit both the individual and those they care about.

<u>WHAT DO WE NOW KNOW</u> ABOUT GENUINELY CARING USING PATIENCE?

HOW PATIENT ARE YOU IN CARING FOR OTHERS?
QUIZ

Instructions: Answer each question honestly based on your typical behavior. At the end, tally your points to see how patience influences your care for others!

1. **A friend is venting about a bad day. You:**
   - o   A. Listen attentively without interrupting, offering support. (3 points)
   - o   B. Listen but occasionally check your watch or phone. (2 points)
   - o   C. Interrupt with advice or change the topic. (1 point)
2. **Your child or younger sibling is struggling with homework. You:**
   - o   A. Sit with them patiently and help them understand. (3 points)
   - o   B. Help them for a while but get frustrated if they don't get it. (2 points)
   - o   C. Tell them to figure it out on their own. (1 point)
3. **A colleague is learning a new task and makes several mistakes. You:**
   - o   A. Patiently guide them through the process again. (3 points)
   - o   B. Correct them but show signs of impatience. (2 points)
   - o   C. Take over the task to get it done quickly. (1 point)
4. **You're stuck in traffic with a friend who is late for an important meeting. You:**
   - o   A. Stay calm and reassure them it will be okay. (3 points)

- o B. Express mild frustration but try to stay positive. (2 points)
- o C. Complain and stress out, making them more anxious. (1 point)

5. **A family member repeatedly asks for help with a simple task. You:**
    - o A. Help them each time with patience and a smile. (3 points)
    - o B. Help them but suggest they try to remember how to do it. (2 points)
    - o C. Show frustration and tell them to figure it out. (1 point)

6. **In a group project, one member is slow to contribute. You:**
    - o A. Encourage them and offer help to get them up to speed. (3 points)
    - o B. Wait for them but start getting annoyed. (2 points)
    - o C. Do the work yourself and exclude them from the process. (1 point)

7. **You're teaching someone a new skill. They don't catch on quickly. You:**
    - o A. Break down the steps and patiently explain again. (3 points)
    - o B. Explain again but with less enthusiasm. (2 points)
    - o C. Show frustration and move on without them. (1 point)

8. **You're waiting for a friend who is running late. You:**
    - o A. Use the time to relax or do something productive. (3 points)
    - o B. Wait but frequently check the time and feel irritated. (2 points)
    - o C. Call them to express your annoyance. (1 point)

9. **A customer or client has many questions about your service/product. You:**
    - o   A. Answer all their questions patiently and thoroughly. (3 points)
    - o   B. Answer their questions but try to hurry them along. (2 points)
    - o   C. Show impatience and cut the conversation short. (1 point)
10. **Your friend is indecisive about what to order at a restaurant. You:**
    - o   A. Wait patiently while they make their decision. (3 points)
    - o   B. Offer suggestions to speed up the process. (2 points)
    - o   C. Show irritation and urge them to hurry up. (1 point)

Scoring:

- **25-30 points**: You are very patient and genuinely care for others. Your patience helps build strong, trusting relationships.
- **18-24 points**: You show patience but can improve. Focus on staying calm and supportive, even in frustrating situations.
- **10-17 points**: Your patience is limited. Reflect on how being more patient can improve your interactions and relationships.
- **0-9 points**: Patience is not your strong suit. Consider the benefits of patience and practice staying calm and supportive.

Reflection: Based on your score, think about areas where you can enhance your patience. Practice active listening, stay calm in stressful situations, and offer support without frustration. Patience can strengthen your relationships and lead to a more fulfilling and supportive life.

GENUINELY CARING

POWER #9 – COMPASSION

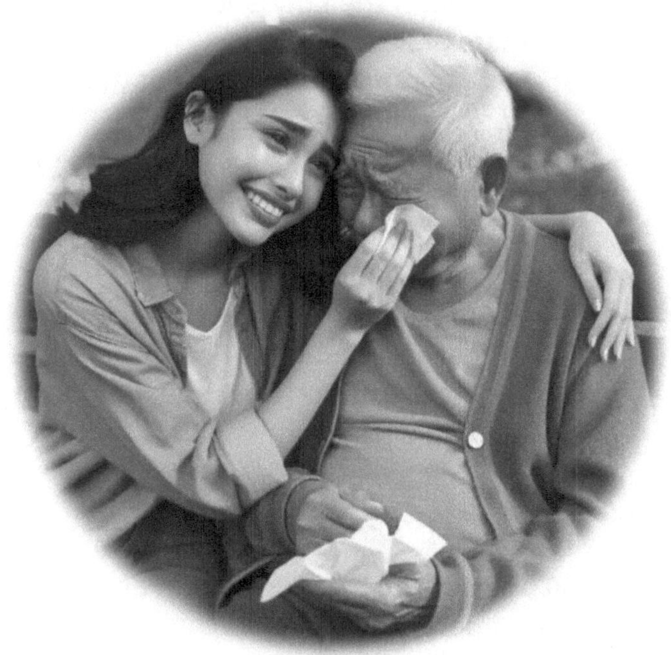

Developing compassion involves nurturing empathy, understanding, and kindness towards others. Here are some effective ways to cultivate compassion:

PRACTICE MINDFULNESS AND MEDITATION

- Loving-Kindness Meditation (Metta): This meditation practice focuses on developing feelings of goodwill and compassion towards oneself and others.
- Mindfulness: Being present in the moment helps you become more aware of your own and others' emotions, fostering a compassionate mindset.

UNDERSTAND AND SHARE FEELINGS

- Empathy: Put yourself in others' shoes to understand their feelings and perspectives. This can help you respond with compassion.
- Active Listening: Truly listen to what others are saying without interrupting or judging. This shows that you care and are willing to understand their experiences.

EDUCATE YOURSELF

- Read about Different Experiences: Learn about the lives and challenges of people from different backgrounds and cultures. This can broaden your perspective and increase your compassion.
- Watch Documentaries and Read Books: Stories and documentaries about others' lives can provide deep insights into their struggles and triumphs.

PRACTICE SELF-COMPASSION

- Be Kind to Yourself: Treat yourself with the same kindness and understanding that you would offer a friend. This helps you extend compassion to others.
- Recognize Common Humanity: Understand that everyone makes mistakes and experiences pain. This can help you be more forgiving and compassionate towards yourself and others.

ENGAGE IN ACTS OF KINDNESS

- Volunteer: Helping others through volunteer work can foster a sense of compassion and empathy.
- Random Acts of Kindness: Small acts, like holding the door open for someone or offering a

compliment, can make a big difference and cultivate a compassionate attitude.

REFLECT ON YOUR ACTIONS AND EMOTIONS

- Journaling: Write about your experiences, thoughts, and feelings. Reflect on how you can be more compassionate in different situations.
- Daily Reflection: Spend a few minutes each day reflecting on how you interacted with others and consider ways to be more compassionate.

CONNECT WITH OTHERS

- Build Strong Relationships: Deep, meaningful relationships can help you understand and care for others more deeply.
- Join Support Groups: Being part of a group with shared experiences can foster a sense of community and compassion.

CULTIVATE GRATITUDE

- Gratitude Journaling: Regularly note things you are grateful for. This can shift your focus from negativity to positivity, making it easier to be compassionate.
- Express Gratitude: Thank others for their kindness and support, which can foster a compassionate mindset.

LEARN FROM ROLE MODELS

- Study Compassionate Figures: Look up to individuals known for their compassion, such as Mother Teresa, the Dalai Lama, or local community leaders.

- Mentorship: Find a mentor who embodies compassion and learn from their behavior and approach to life.

PRACTICE PATIENCE

- **Develop Patience**: Being patient with others allows you to respond with understanding and kindness rather than frustration.
- **Mindful Breathing**: When you feel impatience rising, take deep breaths to calm yourself and approach the situation with compassion.

EMBRACE VULNERABILITY

- Share Your Own Struggles: Being open about your challenges can create deeper connections and mutual compassion.
- Be Open to Others' Vulnerability: Encourage and support others to share their feelings and experiences without judgment.

Developing compassion is a continuous journey that requires practice and commitment. By incorporating these strategies into your daily life, you can cultivate a more compassionate mindset and positively impact those around you.

WHAT COMPASSION STRATEGY OR STRATEGIES SEEM MOST ATTRACTIVE TO **YOU** THAT WILL MAKE THE MOST IMPACT IN YOUR LIFE RIGHT NOW?

1.____________________________________

2.____________________________________

3.____________________________________

WHY WOULD THIS STRATEGY OR STRATEGIES MAKE THE MOST IMPACT IN YOUR LIFE RIGHT NOW?

1.____________________________________

____

WHAT **STUDIES** SHOW THE BENEFITS OF GENUINELY CARING FOR OTHERS USING COMPASSION?

Several studies highlight the benefits of genuinely caring about others using compassion. These benefits span psychological, physical, and social domains. Here are some key studies and their findings:

COMPASSION AND PSYCHOLOGICAL WELL-BEING

- Study: A study published in the *Journal of Clinical Psychology* examined the relationship between compassion and psychological well-being.
- Findings: The researchers found that individuals who regularly practiced compassion towards others experienced lower levels of anxiety and depression. Compassionate individuals also reported higher levels of overall life satisfaction and happiness.

COMPASSION AND PHYSICAL HEALTH

- Study: Research published in the *Health Psychology* journal explored the effects of compassion on physical health.
- Findings: The study found that individuals who engaged in compassionate behaviors had lower levels of inflammation and better immune function. This suggests that compassion can have tangible benefits for physical health, possibly due to reduced stress levels.

COMPASSION AND SOCIAL CONNECTION

- Study: A study in the *Journal of Social Psychology* investigated the impact of compassion on social relationships.
- Findings: The study found that compassionate individuals were more likely to form strong, positive relationships. They were also more likely to be perceived as trustworthy and supportive, which enhances social bonds and networks.

COMPASSION AND PROFESSIONAL SUCCESS

- Study: Research in the *Journal of Organizational Behavior* examined the role of compassion in the workplace.
- Findings: The study showed that leaders who demonstrated compassion were more effective in their roles. Compassionate leadership was associated with higher employee satisfaction, reduced turnover, and improved team performance.

NEUROSCIENCE OF COMPASSION

- Study: A study published in *Social Cognitive and Affective Neuroscience* explored the neural correlates of compassion.
- Findings: The researchers found that practicing compassion activates brain regions associated with reward and positive emotions. This neural activation can lead to increased feelings of happiness and well-being.

COMPASSION AND ALTRUISM

- Study: Research published in the *Journal of Personality and Social Psychology* investigated the link between compassion and altruistic behavior.

- Findings: The study found that individuals who cultivated compassion were more likely to engage in altruistic behaviors, such as helping others and volunteering. This not only benefits recipients but also enhances the giver's sense of purpose and fulfillment.

COMPASSION AND RESILIENCE

- Study: A study in the *Journal of Positive Psychology* explored how compassion affects resilience.
- Findings: The researchers found that individuals who practiced self-compassion and compassion towards others were more resilient in the face of adversity. They were better able to cope with stress and recover from setbacks.

These studies collectively demonstrate that compassion is beneficial not only for those who receive it but also for those who practice it. By fostering positive emotions, enhancing social connections, improving physical health, and increasing resilience, compassion can significantly enhance overall well-being and quality of life.

<u>**WHAT DO WE NOW KNOW**</u> ABOUT GENUINELY CARING USING COMPASSION?

HOW COMPASSIONATE ARE YOU? QUIZ

Instructions: Answer each question honestly based on your typical behavior. At the end, tally your points to see how compassion influences your care for others!

1. **A friend is feeling down and confides in you. You:**
   - o A. Listen attentively and offer words of comfort and support. (3 points)
   - o B. Listen but quickly offer solutions to their problems. (2 points)
   - o C. Change the subject to something more positive. (1 point)
2. **You see someone struggling with heavy bags. You:**
   - o A. Offer to help carry the bags to their destination. (3 points)
   - o B. Encourage them verbally but don't physically help. (2 points)
   - o C. Walk by and hope someone else helps them. (1 point)
3. **A colleague is overwhelmed with work. You:**
   - o A. Offer to assist them with some of their tasks. (3 points)
   - o B. Sympathize with them but focus on your own work. (2 points)
   - o C. Assume they can handle it and do nothing. (1 point)
4. **You notice a stranger crying in public. You:**
   - o A. Approach them and ask if they need any help. (3 points)
   - o B. Feel bad for them but keep your distance. (2 points)

5. **A friend is sick and unable to cook for themselves. You:**
   - o A. Cook a meal and bring it to them. (3 points)
   - o B. Offer to order them food delivery. (2 points)
   - o C. Suggest they call a delivery service. (1 point)
6. **You hear about a community member losing their home to a fire. You:**
   - o A. Organize a fundraiser or collection to help them. (3 points)
   - o B. Donate money or items but don't get involved further. (2 points)
   - o C. Feel sorry for them but don't take any action. (1 point)
7. **A friend is nervous about an upcoming exam. You:**
   - o A. Offer to help them study and reassure them. (3 points)
   - o B. Wish them luck and tell them they'll do fine. (2 points)
   - o C. Tell them everyone gets nervous and they should just relax. (1 point)
8. **You see a homeless person asking for food. You:**
   - o A. Buy them a meal or give them food you have. (3 points)
   - o B. Give them a small amount of money. (2 points)
   - o C. Avoid eye contact and walk past them. (1 point)
9. **A friend is going through a breakup. You:**
   - o A. Spend time with them, listen, and offer emotional support. (3 points)

- B. Check in on them occasionally to see how they are doing. (2 points)
  - C. Give them space and hope they get through it on their own. (1 point)
10. **You notice your neighbor struggling with yard work. You:**
    - A. Offer to help them with the work. (3 points)
    - B. Offer them advice on how to make it easier. (2 points)
    - C. Continue with your own tasks without offering help. (1 point)

Scoring:

- **25-30 points**: You are very compassionate and genuinely care for others. Your compassion helps build strong, supportive relationships and makes you a valued friend and community member.
- **18-24 points**: You show compassion but can improve. Focus on taking more proactive steps to help and support others.
- **10-17 points**: Your compassion is somewhat lacking. Reflect on how you can be more compassionate in your interactions and relationships.
- **0-9 points**: Compassion is not a strong suit for you. Consider the benefits of compassion and how adopting a more compassionate attitude can improve your relationships and personal growth.

Reflection: Based on your score, think about areas where you can enhance your compassion. Practice active listening, offer help proactively, and be more present in the lives of those around you.

GENUINELY CARING

POWER #10 – ENCOURAGEMENT

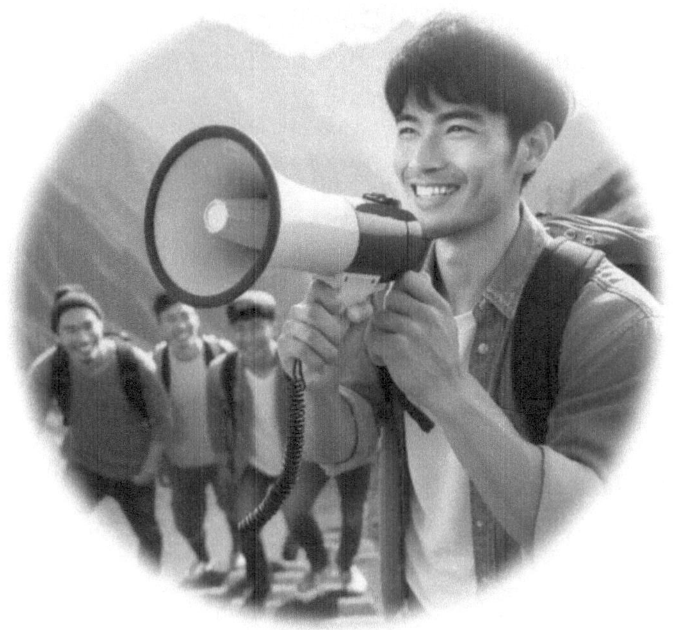

Developing encouragement involves nurturing a positive attitude, being supportive, and actively uplifting others. Here are some effective ways to become more encouraging:

PRACTICE POSITIVE AFFIRMATIONS

- Daily Affirmations: Start your day with positive affirmations to boost your own confidence and positivity. This can make it easier to encourage others.
- Affirm Others: Regularly offer genuine compliments and acknowledge others' strengths and achievements.

LISTEN ACTIVELY

- Show Genuine Interest: Pay close attention to what others are saying without interrupting. This shows that you value their thoughts and feelings.
- Ask Open-Ended Questions: Encourage others to share more by asking questions that require more than yes or no answers.

BE EMPATHETIC

- Understand Feelings: Try to understand others' emotions and perspectives. This empathy can help you offer more meaningful and supportive encouragement.
- Validate Emotions: Acknowledge and validate the feelings of others, letting them know it's okay to feel the way they do.

OFFER SPECIFIC PRAISE

- Highlight Specific Achievements: Instead of general praise, focus on specific actions or accomplishments. This makes your encouragement more meaningful and impactful.
- Celebrate Progress: Acknowledge even small steps towards a goal, as recognizing progress can be very motivating.

BE POSITIVE AND OPTIMISTIC

- Focus on Solutions: When discussing challenges, steer the conversation towards possible solutions and positive outcomes.
- Share Optimism: Express a hopeful outlook about future possibilities, which can inspire and uplift others.

MODEL ENCOURAGING BEHAVIOR

- Lead by Example: Demonstrate encouraging behavior in your actions. Show others how to be supportive and positive through your own conduct.
- Stay Positive in Adversity: Show resilience and optimism in difficult situations, providing a model for others to emulate.

PROVIDE CONSTRUCTIVE FEEDBACK

- Be Constructive: When offering feedback, focus on how someone can improve rather than just pointing out what went wrong.
- Balance Criticism with Praise: Ensure that any constructive criticism is balanced with positive feedback to keep the overall tone encouraging.

SUPPORT OTHERS' GOALS

- Be a Cheerleader: Actively support and cheer on others in their pursuits and goals. Show enthusiasm for their progress and achievements.
- Offer Help: Provide assistance or resources to help others achieve their goals.

CREATE A POSITIVE ENVIRONMENT

- Foster Positivity: Create an environment, whether at home, work, or in social settings, where positive interactions are the norm.
- Encourage Teamwork: Promote a culture of collaboration and mutual support.

USE ENCOURAGING LANGUAGE

- Choose Words Carefully: Use language that is uplifting and positive. Avoid negative or discouraging phrases.
- Be Inclusive: Use inclusive language that makes everyone feel valued and supported.

PRACTICE PATIENCE

- Be Patient with Others: Understand that growth and progress take time. Encourage others to be patient with themselves as well.
- Show Understanding: Be understanding and supportive during setbacks and challenges.

REFLECT ON ENCOURAGING MOMENTS

- Keep a Journal: Reflect on times when you've successfully encouraged others. Analyze what worked well and how it made you and the other person feel.
- Learn from Others: Observe and learn from individuals who are naturally encouraging. Note their techniques and attitudes.

STAY CONNECTED

- Maintain Relationships: Keep in touch with friends, family, and colleagues. Regular contact helps you stay aware of when others might need encouragement.
- Be Available: Make yourself available to listen and support others when they need it.

By incorporating these practices into your daily life, you can develop a habit of encouragement that positively impacts those around you.

WHAT ENCOURAGEMENT STRATEGY OR STRATEGIES SEEM MOST ATTRACTIVE TO **YOU** THAT WILL MAKE THE MOST IMPACT IN YOUR LIFE RIGHT NOW?

1.____

2.____

3.____

WHY WOULD THIS STRATEGY OR STRATEGIES MAKE THE MOST IMPACT IN YOUR LIFE RIGHT NOW?

1.____

____

WHAT **STUDIES** SHOW THE BENEFITS OF GENUINELY CARING FOR OTHERS USING ENCOURAGEMENT?

Several studies highlight the benefits of genuinely caring about others using encouragement. These benefits encompass improved psychological well-being, enhanced performance, and strengthened relationships. Here are some key studies and their findings:

ENCOURAGEMENT AND ACADEMIC PERFORMANCE

Study: Research published in the *Journal of Educational Psychology* examined the impact of teacher encouragement on student performance.

Findings: The study found that students who received regular encouragement from teachers demonstrated higher academic performance and greater motivation to learn. Encouragement was linked to increased self-efficacy and a positive attitude towards learning.

ENCOURAGEMENT IN THE WORKPLACE

Study: A study in the *Journal of Applied Psychology* explored the effects of managerial encouragement on employee performance.

Findings: The research revealed that employees who received encouragement from their managers were more engaged, showed higher job satisfaction, and were more productive. Encouragement also reduced turnover rates and increased organizational commitment.

ENCOURAGEMENT AND MENTAL HEALTH

Study: A study published in *Behavior Research and Therapy* investigated the relationship between social support, encouragement, and mental health.

Findings: The study found that individuals who received encouragement from their social networks experienced lower levels of anxiety and depression. Encouragement provided emotional support, reducing stress and enhancing overall mental health.

ENCOURAGEMENT AND PHYSICAL HEALTH

Study: Research in the *Health Psychology* journal examined the impact of social encouragement on health behaviors.

Findings: The study showed that individuals who received encouragement to adopt healthy behaviors, such as exercising or quitting smoking, were more likely to succeed. Encouragement acted as a motivational factor, leading to better physical health outcomes.

ENCOURAGEMENT AND CHILD DEVELOPMENT

Study: A study in the *Journal of Child Psychology and Psychiatry* explored the effects of parental encouragement on child development.

Findings: The research indicated that children who received consistent encouragement from their parents showed better emotional and social development. Encouragement was associated with higher self-esteem and better peer relationships.

ENCOURAGEMENT AND RELATIONSHIP QUALITY

Study: A study published in the *Journal of Social and Personal Relationships* examined the role of encouragement in romantic relationships.

Findings: The study found that couples who regularly encouraged each other reported higher relationship satisfaction and stronger emotional bonds. Encouragement fostered trust, mutual support, and a sense of partnership.

ENCOURAGEMENT AND TEAM PERFORMANCE

Study: Research in the *Journal of Organizational Behavior* investigated the impact of peer encouragement on team performance.

Findings: The study revealed that teams where members encouraged each other showed improved collaboration, creativity, and overall performance. Encouragement enhanced team cohesion and collective problem-solving abilities.

These studies collectively demonstrate that encouragement plays a crucial role in enhancing various aspects of life, including academic achievement, workplace performance, mental and physical health, child development, relationship quality, and team dynamics. By fostering a supportive and positive environment, encouragement helps individuals and groups thrive, leading to better outcomes and improved well-being for all involved.

<u>WHAT DO WE NOW KNOW</u> ABOUT GENUINELY CARING USING ENCOURAGEMENT?

HOW ENCOURAGING ARE YOU? QUIZ

Instructions: Answer each question honestly based on your typical behavior. At the end, tally your points to see how your encouragement influences your care for others!

1. **A friend shares their new business idea with you. You:**
   - o A. Show excitement, offer praise, and ask how you can help. (3 points)
   - o B. Say it sounds interesting and wish them good luck. (2 points)
   - o C. Point out potential challenges and risks right away. (1 point)
2. **A colleague is nervous about giving a presentation. You:**
   - o A. Reassure them they'll do great and offer to help them practice. (3 points)
   - o B. Tell them not to worry and that they'll be fine. (2 points)
   - o C. Say everyone gets nervous and it's no big deal. (1 point)
3. **A family member wants to pursue a new hobby. You:**
   - o A. Encourage them to go for it and offer your support. (3 points)
   - o B. Tell them it's a good idea if they have the time. (2 points)
   - o C. Question if they really have the time and energy for it. (1 point)
4. **Your friend is trying to get back into shape. You:**

- o A. Cheer them on, offer to join them in workouts, and celebrate their progress. (3 points)
  - o B. Support them verbally and check in occasionally. (2 points)
  - o C. Say it's tough but they should stick to it. (1 point)

5. **A colleague is considering applying for a promotion. You:**
   - o A. Encourage them wholeheartedly and help them prepare their application. (3 points)
   - o B. Say it's worth a try and offer basic advice. (2 points)
   - o C. Mention how competitive it will be and wish them luck. (1 point)

6. **A friend is dealing with a personal setback. You:**
   - o A. Offer words of encouragement and help them see the positives. (3 points)
   - o B. Tell them things will get better soon. (2 points)
   - o C. Suggest they move on and focus on other things. (1 point)

7. **Your child or sibling is learning a new skill. You:**
   - o A. Praise their efforts and progress and help them when needed. (3 points)
   - o B. Encourage them but let them figure it out on their own. (2 points)
   - o C. Point out what they're doing wrong to help them improve. (1 point)

8. **A friend is feeling unmotivated about their goals. You:**
   - o A. Help them set small, achievable steps and cheer them on. (3 points)

- o B. Remind them of why they started and tell them to keep going. (2 points)
- o C. Suggest they take a break and come back to it later. (1 point)

9. **A coworker is struggling with a new project. You:**
   - o A. Offer your assistance and encourage them to keep trying. (3 points)
   - o B. Give them some tips and wish them luck. (2 points)
   - o C. Tell them it's okay to ask someone else for help. (1 point)

10. **Your friend wants to participate in a challenging event (e.g., a marathon). You:**
    - o A. Cheer them on, help them train, and offer constant support. (3 points)
    - o B. Encourage them and offer to be there on the day of the event. (2 points)
    - o C. Express doubt about whether they're ready but wish them luck. (1 point)

Scoring:

- **25-30 points**: You are very encouraging and genuinely care for others. Your positive reinforcement helps build strong, supportive relationships and motivates those around you.
- **18-24 points**: You show encouragement but can improve. Focus on being more proactive in offering support and celebrating others' efforts.
- **10-17 points**: Your encouragement is somewhat lacking. Reflect on how you can be more uplifting in your interactions and relationships.
- **0-9 points**: Encouragement is not a strong suit for you. Consider the benefits of encouragement and how adopting a more supportive attitude

can improve your relationships and personal growth.

Reflection: Based on your score, think about areas where you can enhance your encouragement. Practice celebrating others' efforts, offering help proactively, and being a positive influence in their lives. Encouragement can strengthen your relationships and lead to a more fulfilling and supportive life.

PART 3

SUSTAINING THE POWER

MINDSET SHIFTS

WHAT **MINDSET SHIFTS** ARE NECESSARY FOR GENUINELY CARING ABOUT OTHERS?

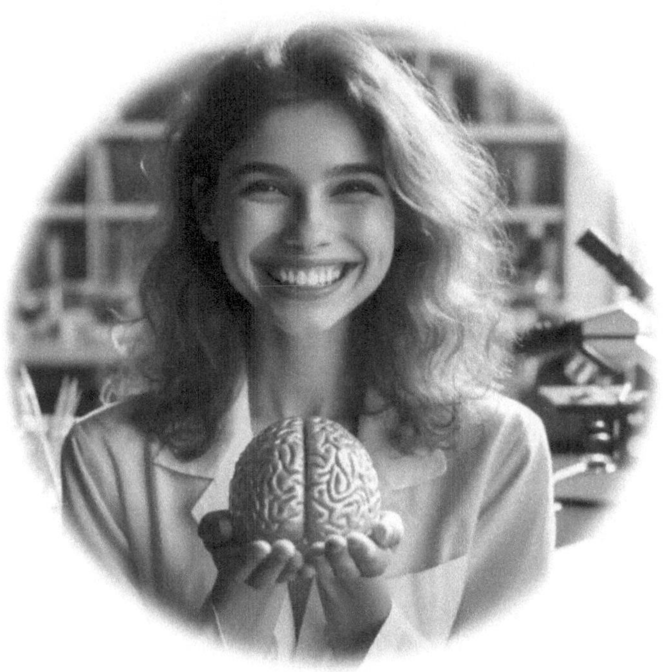

To genuinely start caring about others, several mindset shifts can be beneficial. These shifts involve cultivating attitudes and perspectives that prioritize empathy, compassion, and the well-being of others. Here are some key mindset shifts that can help foster genuine care:

SHIFT FROM SELF-CENTEREDNESS TO EMPATHY:

Mindset Shift: Recognize that others have their own perspectives, experiences, and emotions that are equally valid and important as your own. Empathy involves actively trying to understand and share the feelings of others, which can shift the focus away from oneself towards the needs and experiences of others.

SHIFT FROM INDIFFERENCE TO COMPASSION:

Mindset Shift: Develop a mindset of compassion, which involves feeling concern for the suffering and well-being of others. Understand that everyone faces challenges and struggles, and approach interactions with kindness and a desire to alleviate others' pain or difficulties.

SHIFT FROM JUDGMENT TO ACCEPTANCE:

Mindset Shift: Practice non-judgmental acceptance of others. Recognize that everyone is on their own journey with unique strengths and weaknesses. Avoid making quick judgments or assumptions, and instead, strive to appreciate and respect the diversity of human experiences.

SHIFT FROM ISOLATION TO CONNECTION:

Mindset Shift: Embrace the importance of social connections and community. Recognize that caring for others builds meaningful relationships and strengthens social bonds. Shift from a mindset of isolation or independence to one that values interdependence and mutual support.

SHIFT FROM TRANSACTIONAL TO RELATIONAL:

Mindset Shift: View relationships as opportunities for genuine connection and mutual growth, rather than purely transactional interactions. Approach interactions with authenticity, sincerity, and a willingness to invest in the well-being of others without expecting immediate returns.

SHIFT FROM FIXED TO GROWTH MINDSET:

Mindset Shift: Adopt a growth mindset that believes in the potential for personal and interpersonal growth. Recognize that caring for others is a skill that can be developed and strengthened over time through practice, learning, and reflection.

SHIFT FROM FEAR TO COURAGE:

Mindset Shift: Overcome fears of vulnerability, rejection, or discomfort that may prevent genuine care. Cultivate courage to step outside your comfort zone, reach out to others, and offer support even in challenging or uncertain situations.

SHIFT FROM COMPETITION TO COLLABORATION:

Mindset Shift: Embrace a mindset of collaboration and cooperation rather than competition. Recognize that supporting others and working together towards common goals can lead to collective success and positive outcomes for everyone involved.

SHIFT FROM INSTANT GRATIFICATION TO LONG-TERM IMPACT:

Mindset Shift: Value the long-term impact of caring for others over immediate rewards or gratification. Understand that genuine care often involves sustained effort, patience, and investment in building lasting relationships and contributing to the well-being of others.

SHIFT FROM INDIVIDUALISM TO COLLECTIVE RESPONSIBILITY:

Mindset Shift: Embrace a sense of collective responsibility for the well-being of others and the community. Recognize that everyone has a role to play in creating a supportive and compassionate society where individuals can thrive.

These mindset shifts can help individuals cultivate a genuine caring attitude towards others, fostering deeper connections, personal growth, and a positive impact on their communities and beyond.

MINDSET REFLECTION

WHAT ARE SOME GREAT QUESTIONS ABOUT MINDSET SHIFTS FOR GENUINELY CARING?

IDENTIFY A LIMITING BELIEF:

What is one belief you hold that may be limiting your ability to genuinely care for others? Why do you think you hold this belief?

____

____

How can you reframe this belief to foster greater empathy and compassion?

____

____

REFLECT ON PAST EXPERIENCES:

Think of a time when you felt genuinely cared for by someone else. How did their actions and attitude impact you?

____

____

How can you incorporate those behaviors into your interactions with others?

____

____

EMPATHY DEVELOPMENT:

Reflect on a recent interaction where you felt disconnected or indifferent. What could you have done differently to show genuine care?

____

____

How can you practice active listening and empathy in future interactions?

____

____

RECOGNIZE COMMON HUMANITY:

Write about a person you find difficult to care for. What common human experiences or emotions do you share with this person?

____

____

How can recognizing these shared experiences help you develop a more compassionate attitude towards them?

____

____

CHALLENGE JUDGMENTS:

Reflect on a time when you judged someone harshly. What assumptions did you make about them?

____

____

How can you challenge these assumptions and approach similar situations with an open and caring mindset?

____

____

PRACTICE GRATITUDE:

List three people in your life who have shown you kindness and care. How did their actions influence your well-being?

____

____

How can you express gratitude for their care and extend similar kindness to others?

____

____

VISUALIZE POSITIVE OUTCOMES:

Imagine a future scenario where you show genuine care for someone in need. What actions do you take, and how do they respond?

____

____

How does this positive outcome make you feel, and what steps can you take to make it a reality?

____

____

SELF-COMPASSION:

Reflect on a moment when you were hard on yourself. How did this impact your ability to care for others?

____

____

How can practicing self-compassion improve your capacity to show genuine care to others?

____

____

ACTS OF KINDNESS:

Recall a recent act of kindness you performed. How did it make you feel, and what was the response of the person you helped?

____

____

How can you incorporate more small acts of kindness into your daily routine?

____

____

LEARNING FROM ROLE MODELS:

Who is someone you admire for their genuine care and compassion? What specific qualities or actions make them a role model for you?

____

____

How can you emulate these qualities in your own life?

____

____

UNDERSTANDING DIFFERENT PERSPECTIVES:

Write about a situation where you disagreed with someone. How might their perspective be shaped by their experiences and emotions?

____

____

How can understanding their perspective help you approach the situation with more empathy and care?

____

____

COMMIT TO PERSONAL GROWTH:

Identify one area where you want to improve in showing genuine care for others. What specific steps can you take to work on this area?

____

____

How will you measure your progress and stay committed to this personal growth?

____

____

CELEBRATE PROGRESS:

Reflect on a recent situation where you successfully demonstrated genuine care for someone. What did you do, and how did it impact them?

____

____

How can you build on this success and continue to grow in your capacity for empathy and compassion?

____

____

MINDFULNESS AND PRESENCE:

Describe a moment when you were fully present with someone, giving them your undivided attention. How did this presence affect your interaction?

____

____

How can you practice mindfulness to enhance your ability to genuinely care for others in future interactions?

____

____

IMPACT OF CARE:

Think about the broader impact of showing genuine care in your community or social circles. How does your care contribute to a positive environment?

____

____

How can you encourage others to adopt a similar caring mindset?

____

____

These prompts are designed to help you explore and shift your mindset towards greater empathy, compassion, and genuine care for others. Regular journaling on these topics can deepen your understanding and commitment to fostering positive relationships and making a meaningful impact.

REFLECTION

WHAT ARE THE BEST **STRATEGIES FOR REFLECTION** ON GENUINELY CARING?

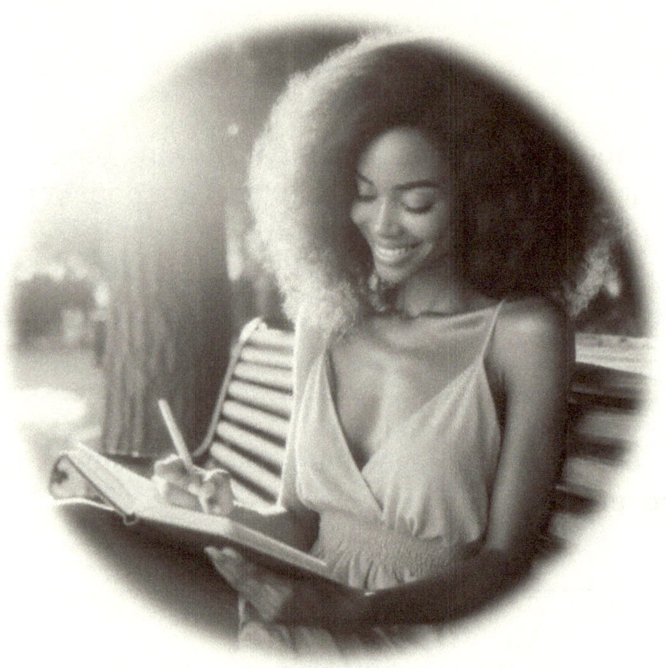

Reflecting on genuinely caring for others involves examining your actions, attitudes, and their impacts on the people around you. Here are some effective strategies for reflection on this important aspect of personal development:

JOURNALING

- Daily Reflection: Write about your daily interactions with others, focusing on moments where you showed care and compassion. Reflect on how these actions affected both you and the other person.

- Specific Prompts: Use prompts such as "How did I show care for someone today?" or "What did I do to make someone feel valued?" to guide your reflections.

MINDFULNESS AND MEDITATION

- Mindful Reflection: Spend time in mindfulness meditation, focusing on your interactions with others. Reflect on your intentions, actions, and the emotional responses of those involved.
- Loving-Kindness Meditation: Practice loving-kindness meditation to cultivate compassion and reflect on how you can extend this care to others.

SELF-ASSESSMENT AND FEEDBACK

- Self-Evaluation: Periodically evaluate your behavior and attitudes towards others. Consider areas where you can improve in showing genuine care.
- Seek Feedback: Ask for feedback from friends, family, or colleagues about how they perceive your caring behaviors. Use this feedback to identify strengths and areas for growth.

GOAL SETTING AND REVIEW

- Set Caring Goals: Set specific goals related to caring for others, such as acts of kindness or supportive behaviors. Review these goals regularly to track your progress.
- Reflect on Achievements: Reflect on the goals you have achieved and how they have impacted your relationships and well-being.

PEER DISCUSSIONS AND SUPPORT GROUPS

- Discussion Groups: Join or form a group where you can discuss experiences and challenges related to caring for others. Learn from others' perspectives and share your own reflections.
- Mentorship: Find a mentor or be a mentor to someone. Reflect on how these relationships enhance your ability to care genuinely.

CASE STUDIES AND SCENARIOS

- Analyze Scenarios: Reflect on specific scenarios where you showed care for others. Analyze what went well and what could be improved.
- Learn from Examples: Study examples of compassionate behavior from others, such as role models or historical figures, and reflect on how you can incorporate similar behaviors into your life.

ARTISTIC AND CREATIVE EXPRESSION

- Creative Journaling: Use art, drawing, or other creative methods to express your reflections on caring for others.
- Storytelling: Write stories or poems about your experiences of caring for others, highlighting the emotions and lessons learned.

REGULAR REFLECTION TIME

- Scheduled Reflection: Dedicate regular time for reflection, whether daily, weekly, or monthly. Consistent reflection helps ingrain the habit and deepen your understanding.
- Quiet Space: Find a quiet, comfortable space where you can reflect without distractions.

REFLECT ON PERSONAL VALUES

- Identify Core Values: Reflect on your core values and how they align with your behaviors towards others. Consider how your actions reflect your commitment to these values.
- Value Alignment: Assess how well your daily actions align with your values of compassion and care.

GRATITUDE PRACTICE

- Gratitude Journaling: Keep a gratitude journal where you note down moments of kindness and care you have given and received. Reflect on how these moments make you feel.
- Express Gratitude: Reflect on how expressing gratitude to others can enhance your relationships and your ability to care genuinely.

VISUALIZATIONS AND MENTAL REHEARSAL

- Visualize Caring Actions: Spend time visualizing scenarios where you can show care and compassion. Mentally rehearse your responses and actions.
- Reflect on Outcomes: After visualizing, reflect on how these caring actions could impact your relationships and your own well-being.

LEARNING FROM CHALLENGES

- Reflect on Difficult Situations: Reflect on situations where it was challenging to show care. Analyze what made it difficult and how you can handle similar situations better in the future.

- **Identify Growth Areas:** Use challenging experiences as opportunities for growth. Reflect on what you learned and how you can improve.

By incorporating these strategies into your routine, you can develop a deeper understanding of your capacity to care for others genuinely, and continually improve your ability to support and uplift those around you.

WHAT **COMMUNITY SUPPORTS SYSTEMS** ARE IN PLACE FOR CONTINUED GROWTH IN GENUINELY CARING FOR OTHERS?

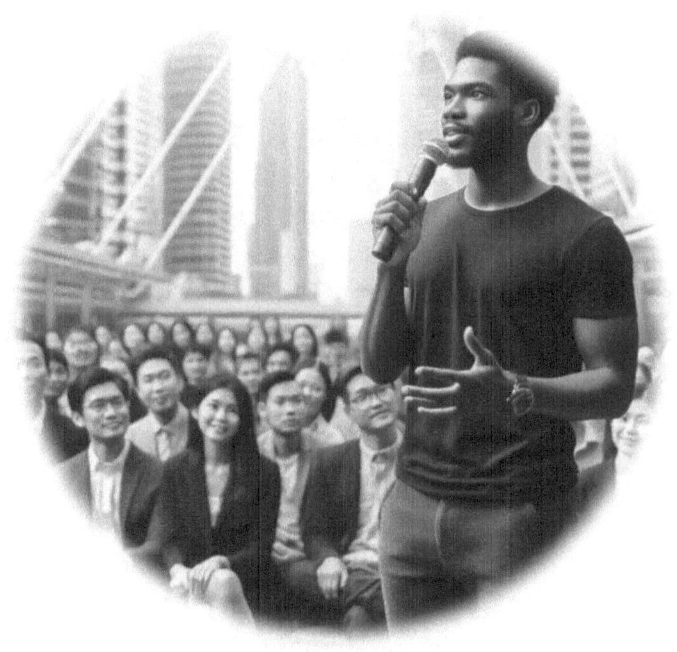

Continued growth in genuinely caring for others can be supported by various community-based systems and resources. These systems often provide opportunities for learning, practice, feedback, and mutual support. Here are several community support systems that can contribute to your ongoing development in this area:

SUPPORT GROUPS AND PEER NETWORKS

- Community Organizations: Join local community organizations or groups focused on volunteering, social justice, or humanitarian efforts. These groups provide opportunities to engage in collective caring activities and learn from others.

- Supportive Networks: Build relationships with like-minded individuals who prioritize compassion and caring. These networks offer emotional support, shared experiences, and encouragement.

MENTORSHIP PROGRAMS

- Mentorship Opportunities: Seek out mentorship programs where experienced individuals guide you in developing your capacity for empathy, compassion, and supportive behaviors.
- Reverse Mentorship: Consider mentoring others, especially in areas where you have strengths. Teaching others can deepen your own understanding and commitment to caring for others.

TRAINING AND WORKSHOPS

- Community Workshops: Attend workshops and training sessions focused on empathy, active listening, conflict resolution, and compassionate communication.
- Skill-Building Programs: Participate in programs that teach practical skills related to caregiving, volunteer management, or community service.

VOLUNTEER OPPORTUNITIES

- Community Service: Engage in volunteer activities that directly involve caring for others, such as serving meals at a shelter, tutoring, or visiting nursing homes.

- Service Projects: Join community service projects that promote empathy and social responsibility, fostering connections with diverse populations.

ONLINE COMMUNITIES AND RESOURCES

- Online Forums and Groups: Participate in online communities focused on empathy, kindness, and social impact. These platforms provide virtual support, discussion forums, and resource sharing.
- Webinars and Virtual Workshops: Attend virtual events that offer insights into compassionate leadership, community building, and effective caregiving practices.

CIVIC ENGAGEMENT AND ADVOCACY

- Advocacy Groups: Get involved in advocacy groups that promote social justice, human rights, and compassionate policies. Participate in campaigns that advocate for marginalized communities and promote empathy in society.
- Community Leadership: Take on leadership roles within community organizations or initiatives that prioritize caring for others, fostering a culture of empathy and support.

EDUCATIONAL INSTITUTIONS

- School-Based Programs: Participate in school-based programs that promote empathy education and peer support initiatives. These programs help cultivate empathy from a young age and encourage lifelong habits of caring.
- University Courses: Take courses or participate in seminars at universities that focus on ethics,

social responsibility, and community engagement.

FAITH-BASED COMMUNITIES

- Faith-Based Organizations: Engage with faith-based communities that emphasize compassion, kindness, and service to others. These communities often provide opportunities for volunteering, social outreach, and spiritual growth.

PEER SUPPORT AND ACCOUNTABILITY

- Accountability Partners: Partner with a friend or colleague who shares your commitment to caring for others. Hold each other accountable for practicing empathy and compassion in daily interactions.
- Peer Coaching: Engage in peer coaching sessions where you provide feedback and support to each other in developing caring behaviors.

PROFESSIONAL DEVELOPMENT PROGRAMS

- Continuing Education: Participate in professional development programs that focus on interpersonal skills, emotional intelligence, and leadership qualities related to caring for others.
- Leadership Development: Take leadership training courses that emphasize compassionate leadership styles and strategies for creating supportive work environments.

COMMUNITY-BASED EVENTS AND GATHERINGS

- Community Gatherings: Attend community events such as forums, discussions, or cultural celebrations that promote unity, understanding, and mutual support.
- Social Activities: Participate in social activities within your community that encourage bonding and foster a sense of belonging and care for others.

PEER-REVIEWED RESEARCH AND PUBLICATIONS

- Stay Informed: Keep up-to-date with peer-reviewed research and publications on topics related to empathy, compassion, and caring behaviors. This knowledge can inform your practices and inspire new ways of caring for others.

SOCIAL MEDIA ENGAGEMENT

- Positive Influences: Follow and engage with social media accounts and platforms that promote kindness, empathy, and community support. Share uplifting stories and resources that inspire others to prioritize caring behaviors.

By actively participating in these community support systems, you can enhance your ability to genuinely care for others, contribute positively to your community, and continue growing in empathy, compassion, and supportive behaviors.

WHAT COMMUNITY SUPPORT SYSTEM(S) STANDS OUT THE MOST FOR **YOU**?

WHAT STANDS OUT MOST ABOUT THIS COMMUNITY SUPPORT SYSTEM OR SYSTEMS THAT YOU'VE SELECTED?

WHO ARE SOME GREAT MENTORS FOR GENUINELY CARING ABOUT OTHERS?

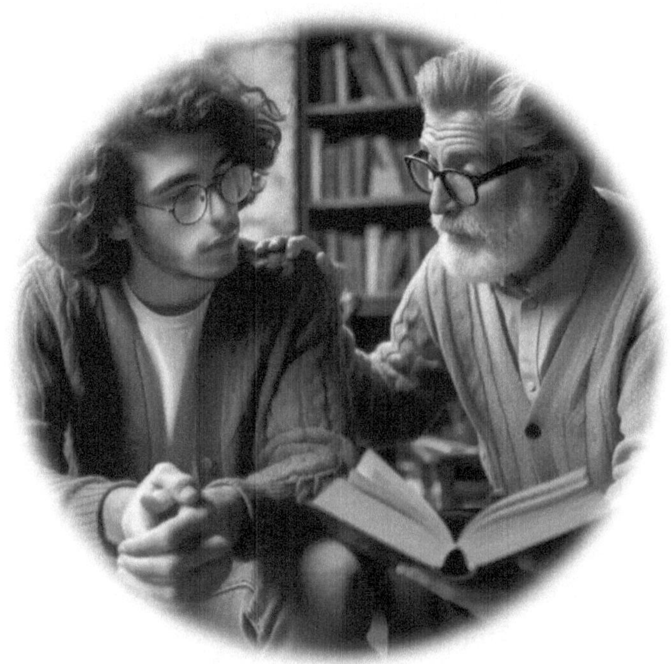

There are several individuals known for their exemplary commitment to genuinely caring about others, serving as inspiring mentors in various fields. Here are a few notable figures who exemplify qualities of empathy, compassion, and altruism:

FRED ROGERS

- Known For: Creator and host of the television program *Mister Rogers' Neighborhood*.
- Legacy: Fred Rogers is remembered for his gentle demeanor, empathy towards children, and messages of kindness and understanding. He promoted the importance of empathy and caring

for others through his television show and advocacy work.

MOTHER TERESA

- Known For: Founder of the Missionaries of Charity, a Roman Catholic congregation dedicated to serving the poor.
- Legacy: Mother Teresa dedicated her life to caring for the sick and impoverished in Calcutta (now Kolkata), India, and around the world. She demonstrated profound compassion and selflessness in her work with the most vulnerable communities.

MAHATMA GANDHI

- Known For: Leader of the Indian independence movement against British rule.
- Legacy: Gandhi advocated for nonviolent resistance and compassion towards all beings. His teachings on empathy, love, and social justice continue to inspire individuals and movements worldwide.

MALALA YOUSAFZAI

- Known For: Pakistani activist for female education and the youngest Nobel Prize laureate.
- Legacy: Malala has shown exceptional courage and compassion in advocating for girls' education and human rights. Despite facing adversity, she continues to inspire others with her commitment to empathy and equality.

DESMOND TUTU

- Known For: South African Anglican bishop and social rights activist.
- Legacy: Desmond Tutu played a key role in the fight against apartheid in South Africa. He is known for his advocacy of nonviolent resistance, reconciliation, and social justice. Tutu's compassionate leadership has left a lasting impact on global human rights movements.

THICH NHAT HANH

- Known For: Vietnamese Buddhist monk, peace activist, and mindfulness teacher.
- Legacy: Thich Nhat Hanh promotes mindfulness, compassion, and peace through his teachings and writings. He emphasizes the importance of living with awareness and cultivating loving-kindness towards oneself and others.

OPRAH WINFREY

- Known For: American media proprietor, talk show host, and philanthropist.
- Legacy: Oprah Winfrey has used her platform to advocate for social issues, education, and personal development. She encourages empathy, self-reflection, and kindness through her humanitarian efforts and media influence.

NELSON MANDELA

- Known For: Anti-apartheid revolutionary and former President of South Africa.
- Legacy: Nelson Mandela exemplified forgiveness, reconciliation, and compassion during and after his imprisonment. His leadership and commitment to equality continue to inspire

efforts towards social justice and human rights globally.

BRENE BROWN

- Known For: Researcher, storyteller, and author focusing on vulnerability, courage, empathy, and shame resilience.
- Legacy: Brene Brown's work emphasizes the importance of empathy, connection, and compassion in fostering meaningful relationships and personal growth. Her insights into vulnerability and empathy have influenced countless individuals and organizations.

DALAI LAMA

- Known For: Spiritual leader of Tibetan Buddhism and advocate for peace and compassion.
- Legacy: The Dalai Lama promotes compassion, forgiveness, and tolerance as essential principles for personal and global well-being. His teachings on empathy and ethical conduct inspire individuals to cultivate kindness and understanding.

These mentors have left enduring legacies through their actions, teachings, and advocacy for genuine care and compassion towards others. Their examples serve as guiding lights for those seeking to deepen their own commitment to empathy and altruism in their lives and communities.

MENTORS

WHO ARE SOME GREAT LOCAL MENTORS?

Finding mentors who exemplify genuine care and compassion can significantly influence your personal growth and community impact. Here are some categories of individuals and specific figures who are often recognized as great mentors in this area:

CATEGORIES OF MENTORS:

Community Leaders: Local leaders who work tirelessly to improve the well-being of their communities through various initiatives and programs.

Nonprofit and NGO Founders: Individuals who have dedicated their lives to causes such as poverty alleviation, education, health, and social justice.

Healthcare Professionals: Doctors, nurses, and mental health professionals who go above and beyond in their care for patients.

Educators: Teachers and professors who invest deeply in the personal and academic growth of their students.

Spiritual Leaders: Pastors, priests, rabbis, imams, and other spiritual guides who provide emotional and spiritual support to their communities.

Social Workers: Professionals dedicated to helping individuals and families in need through direct support and advocacy.

Activists: Individuals who passionately advocate for social change and justice, often at great personal sacrifice.

FINDING LOCAL MENTORS:

Local Nonprofits and Charities: Engage with local organizations and find leaders who inspire you with their dedication to community service.

Community Centers: Attend events and programs at community centers where you can meet and learn from individuals committed to helping others.

Religious Institutions: Connect with spiritual leaders and community members who demonstrate compassion and care.

Educational Institutions: Seek out teachers, counselors, and administrators known for their commitment to student welfare and development.

Healthcare Facilities: Look for healthcare professionals who go above and beyond in patient care and advocacy.

Volunteer Groups: Join local volunteer groups and observe the leaders who organize and motivate others towards charitable activities.

By seeking out and learning from these mentors, you can develop a deeper understanding and practice of genuinely caring for others.

MENTORS

Here's a fun quiz to help you identify and reflect on mentors who exemplify genuine care and compassion. This quiz can also inspire you to seek or become a mentor who positively impacts others.

QUIZ: WHICH GENUINE CARE MENTOR INSPIRES YOU?

1. How do you prefer to show care and support to others?

a) Providing legal assistance and fighting for justice

 b) Offering hands-on help and compassionate care

c) Inspiring and educating through media and storytelling

d) Advocating for education and empowerment

2. What kind of impact do you want to make in your community?

a) Advocate for social justice and equality

b) Help the poor and marginalized

c) Teach kindness and empathy to children

d) Promote education for all, especially girls

3. How do you handle challenges or adversity in your efforts to help others?

a) Fight tirelessly for what is right, despite setbacks

b) Serve with unwavering dedication and humility

c) Use your platform to raise awareness and inspire change

d) Stand up courageously for what you believe in, even at great personal risk

4. Which quality do you admire most in a mentor?

a) Legal expertise and a strong sense of justice

b) Compassionate service and selflessness

c) Ability to connect with and inspire others

d) Courage and dedication to a cause

5. What's your approach to personal growth and learning?

a) Seek out knowledge and continuously educate yourself on social issues

b) Learn through direct service and hands-on experience

c) Embrace creativity and innovation in spreading messages of care

d) Advocate for the rights and education of those in need

6. How do you measure success in your efforts to care for others?

a) Legal victories and policy changes

b) The number of lives positively impacted through direct service

c) The reach and influence of your message

d) Increased access to education and empowerment for marginalized groups

Results:

Mostly A's: Bryan Stevenson

- **Role**: Founder of the Equal Justice Initiative
- **Contribution**: Known for fighting racial injustice and providing legal representation to the wrongly convicted. If you value justice and legal advocacy, Bryan Stevenson is your ideal mentor.

Mostly B's: Mother Teresa (Saint Teresa of Calcutta)

- **Role**: Founder of the Missionaries of Charity
- **Contribution**: Renowned for her work with the poor and sick, embodying compassion and selfless service. If you admire hands-on help and compassionate care, Mother Teresa is your inspiration.

Mostly C's: Fred Rogers

- **Role**: Creator and host of "Mister Rogers' Neighborhood"
- **Contribution**: Taught children about kindness, empathy, and understanding through his television program. If you believe in inspiring others through media and storytelling, Fred Rogers is your mentor.

Mostly D's: Malala Yousafzai

- **Role**: Activist for female education and the youngest Nobel Prize laureate
- **Contribution**: Advocates for the education of girls worldwide. If you are passionate about education and empowerment, Malala Yousafzai is your role model.

Reflection:

- **Bryan Stevenson**: Reflect on ways you can advocate for justice in your community. How can you support those who are unfairly treated?
- **Mother Teresa**: Think about how you can offer direct service to those in need. What small acts of kindness can you perform daily?
- **Fred Rogers**: Consider how you can use your talents to spread messages of kindness and empathy. How can you inspire others through your actions and words?
- **Malala Yousafzai**: Reflect on the importance of education and empowerment. How can you support and advocate for equal access to education in your community?

This quiz is designed to be fun and insightful, helping you identify mentors who reflect genuine care and inspire you to make a positive impact in your community. Enjoy reflecting on the qualities you admire and how you can incorporate them into your own life.

CONCLUSION

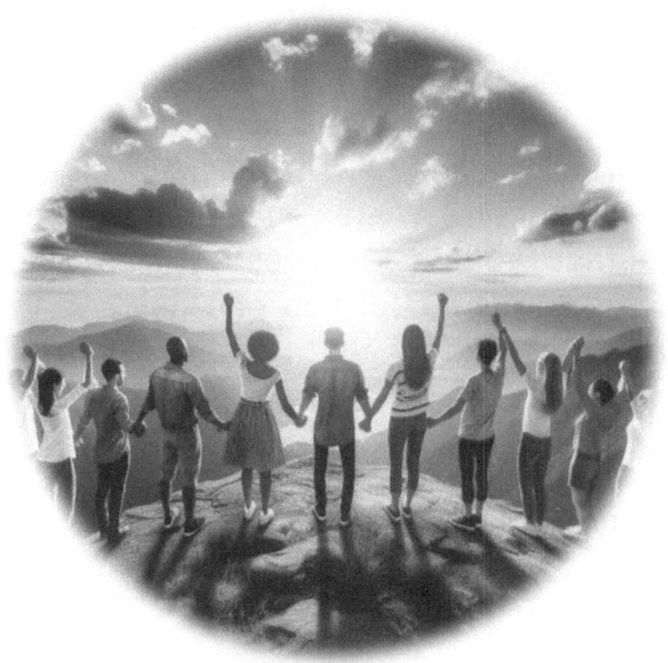

Genuinely caring for others enriches lives, strengthens communities, and fosters a more compassionate, just, and resilient world. Embracing empathy, kindness, and compassion not only benefits individuals but also contributes to the collective well-being and harmonious coexistence of humanity.

THANK YOU GREATLY!

I want to thank you from the bottom of my heart for deciding to better yourself, the community and the world! I'd also like to thank you for supporting me and this message, by picking up this book! I hope it helps enlighten, inspire, and encourage you, as it does me! I would be honored to sign it for you one day and in the meanwhile look forward to your review; as it will help the spread The Power of Genuinely Caring, to help inspire me and others!

I greatly appreciate you!

Cheers,

Isaiah Ward

THE AUTHOR

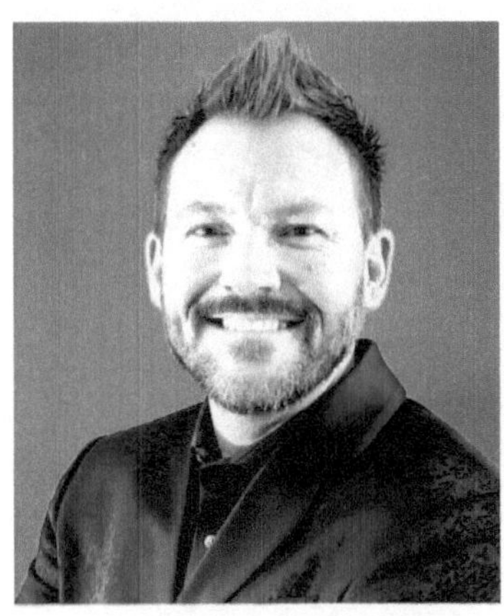

Isaiah Ward changed his life at the age of 18 when he got into direct sales, selling Kirby vacuums door-to-door. He rapidly moved up in the company within 90 days and began travelling throughout the Western United States, helping 1000's of women and men of all ages, 18 and up; thrive in and out of business, applying people skills. The #1 message and strategy for success that he teaches is Genuinely Caring for people. He also became a Father and Life Partner at the young age of 19. His Son is now 21 years of age and thriving in the movie industry with some of Hollywood's greatest, which Isaiah mainly accredits to Genuinely Caring for others. Isaiah has been a life partner to his Son's Mom for 22 years now and is passionate about constantly growing together and believes by Genuinely Caring for enough people, they will live the life they have always dreamed of.